GW00702702

# A to Z of Health Tips

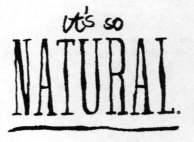

it's so
NATURAL.

## Alan Hayes

SIMON & SCHUSTER
AUSTRALIA

ESSEX COUNTY LIBRARY

A to Z of HEALTH TIPS
First published in Australia in 2002 by
Simon & Schuster (Australia) Pty Limited
20 Barcoo Street, East Roseville NSW 2069

A Viacom Company
Sydney  New York  London

Visit our website at www.simonsaysaustralia.com

© Alan Hayes, 2002

All rights reserved.
No part of this publication may be reproduced,
stored in a retrieval system, or transmitted,
in any form or by any means, electronic, mechanical,
photocopying, recording or otherwise, without
the prior permission of the publisher in writing.

Cataloguing-in-Publication data:

Hayes, Alan.
A to Z of health tips.

ISBN 0731811623

Cover design by Avril Makula
Typeset in 10.5 on 13 Berkeley Book
Printed in Australia by Griffin Press on 79 gsm Bulky Paperback

10 9 8 7 6 5 4 3 2 1

It's So Natural is a registered trade mark
of Alan Hayes and Ernest Berge Phillips.

# Contents

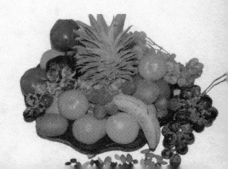

# Author's Note

It must always be remembered that the benefits of herbs, natural foods, correct diet and living foods are cumulative. Instant results do not occur, nor should they be expected.

This book answers many questions for healthy living, but it is not intended to directly or indirectly prescribe the use of the various remedies or dietary changes without the consent of your health practitioner. The intent is only to offer information that you may wish to explore as a natural health alternative. Should you use this information without first obtaining your health practitioner's approval, you are prescribing for yourself. This is your right, but neither I (the author) nor the publisher can assume responsibility for your doing so.

vi

# Introduction

The use of plants for health and as medicines is almost as old as the human race. Ancient races, such as the Egyptians, Greeks and Romans, all used various plants, as did most early civilisations, to ward off evil, treat disease, as medicines, and as tonics and teas. It didn't take long before our ancestors discovered the health-giving properties of various plants.

As knowledge grew, flowers, berries and foliage were all used in the treatment of skin disorders, to vitalise and cleanse hair, and as health treatments. Herbalists were the dispensers of natural remedies, and through experimentation they began to unlock the secrets of the plant world. People turned to them, or the 'Herbals' they wrote, for advice on how to cure or remove every blemish, blotch or spot.

Some herbs were chosen for their special properties. An extract of yarrow was used to suppress skin inflammations, aid skin cleansing, remove dead cells, restrict sebum secretion and help close the pores. Chamomile was used as a soothing agent, while calendula oil was used to clean and soften the skin, and to soothe skin irritations.

One of the most loved and widely used herbs was rosemary. Because of its astringent qualities, it was included in skin tonics, and became a principal ingredient in hair care products.

Other herbs that have an astringent effect are primrose, mint, cowslip, elder and aloe vera. In particular, aloe vera's healing qualities have become well known — its volatile oil contains allantoin, proteins, minerals, vitamins A, B1, B2, C, E and K, and 18 amino acids, all essential in replenishing the body's healing energy.

When bathing became popular, herbs were added to bathwater to relax the body, ease tired and aching muscles and comfort strained nerves. These herbs were chosen for their beneficial properties. For instance, rosemary acted as a sedative; lemon balm and lime flowers treated insomnia.

As you read this book, you will be taken into a world of natural alternatives for health and wellbeing. I'm sure that this book will be rewarding and beneficial.

Alan Hayes

# A to Z of
# Health Tips

# A

## Aches and Pains

Herbs that alleviate pain are meadowsweet and the white willow tree — both are a natural source of aspirin.

Meadowsweet can be taken as a tea to relieve persistent pain, and is available from most health food stores. Take it as directed on the label.

For pain related to a specific ailment or condition, see the alphabetical listing for the ailment or condition.

*See also Aching Joints and Muscles, Chamomile, Muscular Aches and Pains, Witch Hazel Ointment.*

## Aching Joints and Muscles

Add ½ cup of bicarbonate of soda to a hot bath and enjoy a long, relaxing soak. For rheumatic pain add 15 g of crushed fresh ginger or 1 teaspoon of powdered ginger to running bathwater. Don't use any more ginger than recommended, as it can very easily cause burning and reddening of the skin.

Essential oils added to bathwater are also excellent for relieving stiff joints and aching, sore muscles. In the bath, use the following oil combinations:

### Bath Oil for Aching Muscles

*4 drops hyssop essential oil*
*2 drops rosemary essential oil*
*2 drops bay essential oil*
*2 drops rose essential oil*

### *Bath Oil for Stiffness from Sport*

*5 drops hyssop essential oil*
*5 drops rosemary essential oil*
*2 drops bay essential oil*

To ease a hot, painful joint, bind it with a clean, slightly bruised cabbage leaf. Secure firmly in position around the joint with a bandage and leave on overnight.

For temporary relief of muscular aches and pains, blend 6 drops of tea-tree oil with 10 ml of olive oil and apply before and after exercise. To make the oil extra penetrating, add 10 drops of avocado oil to the blend and mix thoroughly. A teaspoon of oil added to a hot bath will also help relieve muscular aches and pains.

*See also Aromatic Shower, Bathing, Chamomile, Joints (Painful), Lavender, Massage, Muscular Aches and Pains, Sprains and Strains, Thyme.*

# Acidity

This is a common complaint, generally caused by diet and excessive alcohol. Whenever discomfort occurs, take either of the following remedies: 1 tablespoon of potato juice in a small glass of warm water before meals; or 1 cup of ginger root tea before meals, or as needed.

Ginger is an excellent natural antacid because it prevents the breakdown of pepsinogen to pepsin; the latter irritates tissue to cause peptic ulcers. Ginger also acts as a catalyst to the pelvic area, and when taken before each meal aids in the elimination of colon gas.

Parsley tea is also helpful in mild cases.

*See also Herbal Teas, Hangover, Indigestion, Jojoba, Medicinal Food, Overindulgence, Thyme, Stomach.*

# Acidophilus

Lactobacilli acidophilus occurs naturally in our bodies and is an inhabitant of our intestines. It works as an intestinal cleanser, and helps prevent fungus, diverticulitis, acne, bad breath, flatulence and constipation. It also helps improve the complexion, relieve fatigue and red eyes, guard against intestinal upsets when on holiday, and aid in the absorption of calcium and other minerals. Acidophilus can also aid in the digestion of milk products, prevent some yeast infections and restore bacterial balance in the intestines, particularly antibiotic-induced diarrhoea.

Acidophilus is essential if you are taking antibiotics, which will destroy friendly intestinal flora and cause an overgrowth of the fungus Monilia abricans. This fungus can grow in the intestines, vagina, lungs, mouth (thrush), on the fingers, or under your fingernails or toenails. However, it will usually disappear after a few days of large amounts of acidophilus culture.

An excellent food source of acidophilus is yogurt, which has long been valued for its therapeutic and nutritional effects. Unfortunately, the amount of acidophilus in yogurt varies widely, so read the label before you buy. A supplement is an effective alternative and is available in tablet, capsule, powder and liquid form.

# Acne

Eating the wrong food and hormonal changes are the main causes of acne. A good diet, incorporating plenty of fresh vegetables — especially celery, parsley, watercress, sprouts, wheat grass and sprouted wheat — fruit and wholegrain foods will get your skin off to a good start. Avoid fried foods, refined flour and sugar, 'junk' food, fats, dairy food and carbonated drinks.

# ACNE CONTROL ROUTINE

▶ Try to avoid too much stress — it can aggravate acne.

▶ Wash 2 or 3 times a day with a glycerine vitamin E soap, or one formulated to deal with oily skin and acne, or cleanse your face with the 'Acne Face Scrub'.

▶ Once a week, deep cleanse with a herbal 'Acne Face Mask'.

▶ After washing or cleansing, rinse your skin with an infusion of chamomile, which is purifying, yarrow, which helps eliminate toxins, and lavender, which is calming and antiseptic.

▶ Dab spots with neat lemon juice to kill germs, cool inflammation and improve blood circulation. If a blemish is coming up, dab on 1 drop of neat lavender oil to help it disappear.

▶ Treat troubled spots and blemishes with a herbal compress.

▶ To help clear blemished facial skin, mix together 2 drops each of lavender and chamomile oil in the palm of your hand, then massage into skin each evening — after thoroughly cleansing your face. Leave on overnight.

▶ Apply calendula ointment to reduce inflammation and improve local healing.

▶ Don't pick at spots — you will spread them and leave scars.

▶ Throw out any dirty make-up. Any make-up puff, sponge or brush that has been touching your face must be thrown out or sterilised.

▶ When using make-up or creams, extract as much as you think you will need and put it onto a clean saucer. Use a clean spatula for extracting creams. At no time touch the contents of any tube or jar, otherwise you will contaminate them. Use the saucer as if it were an artist's palette. When you have finished, throw away any leftover make-up, wipe the saucer clean, and then wash it in hot soapy water.

▶ Use only clean cotton wool to apply make-up. If you use an eye brush, wash it after every use.

▶ Don't let your hair hang over your forehead — it aggravates acne.

▶ Increase your intake of calcium. Dolomite (in tablet or powder form) is excellent, and contains the correct balance of calcium and magnesium.

## BLACKHEADS

After thoroughly cleansing your facial skin, apply a warm compress of parsley, yarrow and lemon grass to the affected area. Steaming is also an excellent way to loosen blackheads while the pores of your skin are open. Prepare your facial vaporiser according to the instructions for *Sinusitis (Inhalant)*, and add 1 drop of lavender oil to the boiling water. Steam your face for 10 minutes.

Rinse your face with hot (but not boiling) water in which you have dissolved 1 teaspoon of apple cider vinegar. Then use two cotton buds to gently, and carefully, push the surrounding skin until the blackhead pops out. Never squeeze blackheads out with your fingernails.

## OCCASIONAL PIMPLES

Occasional pimples are a nuisance, unsightly, and always appear when you least want them to. The following remedy is quick and easy, and will heal a pimple overnight.

Bruise a fresh marigold (*Calendula officinalis*) petal and then gently, but firmly, press it onto the affected spot for 2 to 3 minutes. Repeat this procedure from time to time. (If a fresh flower petal is not available, use a fresh leaf in the same way.)

In the morning there is usually just a trace of redness. This will completely disappear in a few hours if the procedure is repeated one more time.

---

*See also Chamomile, Jojoba, Skin Care.*

# Airborne Bacteria

The disinfectant and antiseptic properties of essential oils can be used in many different ways to help guard your home against airborne bacteria and viruses. In other words, they kill or inhibit the growth of bacteria. When used in an air-spray they can be used throughout the house, but they are particularly effective in the bathroom and toilet, and in a room where someone is ill.

To make a disinfectant and antiseptic air-spray suitable for clearing bacteria and viruses, dissolve 25 drops each of lavender and lemon essential oil and 10 drops of geranium essential oil in 10 ml of methylated spirits, and then blend the mixture with half a litre of distilled water. Store in a plastic pump-spray bottle and use as required on a fine mist setting.

## BURNING ESSENTIAL OILS

Burning essential oils in a simmering pot will also kill airborne bacteria and fungi. Try thyme, lavender, pine or eucalyptus for their fresh fragrance.

A simmering pot is a small ceramic vessel with a candle inside. A saucer containing a mixture of essential oil and water sits on top and the burning candle below releases the oil's fragrant vapours. Add about 10 drops of essential oil to 1 cup of boiling water, preheat the saucer with the candle burning, and then three-quarters fill it with the fragrant water, topping up when required.

# Alcohol

*See Hangover, Overindulgence.*

# Allergies

Why some people develop allergies and others don't remains a medical mystery. The best line of defence in combating them is to remove the offending agent. Of course, we often do not know the cause until specific allergy testing is done, because almost any substance in the world can trigger an allergic reaction. Dairy products, pollens, house dust, pets, wheat, food colorants, preservatives and other additives are common culprits. These can trigger allergic reactions such as asthma, eczema, hyperactivity, fatigue, itching, runny nose, sneezing, headaches, and lumps and bumps.

Seriously consider your diet. Start by avoiding processed, refined 'white foods'; replace these with extra fresh fruit and salads, oats and vegetable juices. Avoid milk and dairy products, tea, coffee, alcohol and carbonated drinks while the attack is on, but drink plenty of filtered or spring water.

Herbs and vitamins will help alleviate the symptoms of allergies. For runny noses and eyes and constant sneezing, horseradish is excellent, as it helps dry up mucus and lessens sensitivity to pollens. Since fresh horseradish can cause a burning sensation when taken on an empty stomach, you may find the tablets (available from health food stores) more acceptable. You should also take plenty of garlic, either in your food or as a tablet; combine this with the horseradish.

Fenugreek seeds, which are good for clearing blocked nasal passages, can be made into a tea. Soak 1 teaspoon of seeds in cold water for 30 minutes, then add boiling water. Allow to infuse, covered, for 10 minutes, then strain and drink.

A cup of alfalfa tea taken 3 times a day during an attack will help give relief. Or blend 10 ml each of honey and apple cider vinegar in a large glass of water. Drink half in the morning and the rest in the evening, about an hour after your meal. For mild to moderate food allergies, drink lots of soda water or 1 teaspoon of bicarbonate of soda dissolved in water.

Include a glass of the following juice blend in your daily morning regime: 200 ml of carrot juice and 150 ml of celery juice, strained through a fine strainer so that it is pulp free. Sip slowly for best digestion.

Chewing a piece of comb honey every day during hay fever attacks often helps to clear the nose and sinuses. If possible, obtain your comb honey from a beekeeper in the area in which you live.

If you have wall-to-wall carpeting, consider going back to timber floors; if you've built on a concrete slab, it's worth considering timber flooring over the top of it. You might also consider sleeping on synthetic pillows — their major advantage (over those made from down) is that you can wash them in hot water.

## STEAM INHALATION

Steam inhalations are also effective for clearing blocked sinuses caused by allergies. Add 1 drop each of pine, eucalyptus and cypress oil to a bowl of hot water, place your face about 30 cm away from the bowl, and drape a towel over your head to form a tent. Do not let the steam escape, do not inhale steam for any longer than 10 minutes, and don't do it more than 3 times a day. (People with heart and blood pressure problems, asthma or other breathing difficulties, broken skin or visible, dilated red veins should avoid using steam inhalations, unless otherwise directed by their health practitioner.)

*See also Hay Fever, Sinusitis.*

# Aloe Vera (*Aloe barbadensis*), The Holy Herb

Aloe vera is one of the oldest medicinal plants in history; according to Hindu legend, it came directly from the Garden of Paradise. The ancient Assyrians, Babylonians, Egyptians and Jews endowed this remarkable plant with holy virtues. For centuries it has been surrounded by folklore about its wide range of benefits and healing powers, and known deservedly as the 'holy herb'.

Aloe vera resembles a cactus, but is actually a perennial succulent which belongs to the lily family. It is the gel in its stiff and fleshy leaves which is used in cosmetics and medicinal preparations: the gel contains 'biogenic stimulators'. Ninety-six per cent of the gel is water, but the remaining 4 per cent includes polysaccharides such as glucose and mannose. These carbohydrates, in conjunction with the water content, moisturise the skin. Other constituents of aloe vera pulp include the natural healer chrysophanic acid, antiseptic saponins, enzymes which combat inflammation, allantoin, minerals, and vitamins A, B1, B2, C, E and K; these all help give this herb unique healing properties. You can grow your own aloe vera plants, or buy the stabilised liquid extract or gel from health food stores.

Of aloe vera's many uses, most probably the best known is in the treatment of burns. Its triple action of pain relief and antiseptic and healing qualities makes this remedy suitable for even serious burns and scalds.

Various other skin conditions will also respond well to aloe vera gel treatment. Tinea ('Athlete's foot') and other fungal infections, and infections of the fingers and toenails should have applications of the gel 2–4 times a day. Superficial cuts, scratches, abrasions, minor burns, stings and bites will heal with the same treatment.

You can make your own aloe vera first aid lotion, suitable for burns (including sunburn), broken skin, scratches and wounds, by blending together 10 ml of glycerine, 12 ml of olive oil, 12 ml of wheat germ oil, 6 drops of calendula essential oil, 20 ml of aloe vera juice or stabilised liquid extract and 45 ml of rosewater. Store in an airtight, amber-coloured glass bottle and shake well before using.

Varicose ulcers will respond to daily applications of aloe vera gel; when spread on the cleaned ulcers it will encourage rapid healing.

As a hair preparation, aloe vera is unequalled. Use it for greasy scalp conditions, dandruff, and as a general hair conditioner, and there will soon be a noticeable improvement. Include 1–2 tablespoons of the liquid extract in your shampoo or massage it directly into your scalp.

The liquid extract can also be used as a mouth rinse, or the gel can be rubbed into the gums, for the treatment of bad breath. Alternatively, brush your teeth and gums with the gel once a week as a precautionary measure.

Taken internally, it is useful for treating digestive disorders, ulcers, colitis, constipation and inflammatory bowel complaints. All internal applications of aloe vera require the advice of your health practitioner.

Aloe vera is easily grown in the home garden, and can be purchased ready to plant out from most nurseries. Make sure that the plant you buy is *Aloe barbadensis* (medicinal aloe), since there are many other varieties which don't have the same healing properties.

---

*See also Burns, Cuts and Abrasions, Dandruff, Fungal Problems, Hair, Oral Hygiene, Skin Irritations, Stings and Bites.*

# Anaemia

Anaemia is a lack of red blood corpuscles. It is generally corrected by adopting a more natural lifestyle, including adequate rest and relaxation and a change of diet.

Include the following foods to ensure both variety and nutrition in your diet: parsley, peas, watercress, barley, cabbage, cauliflower, pumpkin, spinach and tomatoes. If you can be assured that no pesticides have been sprayed on them, also include young dandelion greens and stinging nettles. Chop these up raw and include them in summer salads or lightly steam them and use in winter meals. Other beneficial foods are oranges, apples, apricots, pecan nuts and grapes, when in season (otherwise use raisins).

Drink a small glass of fresh beetroot juice every day or a glass of the following Special Juice Mix.

### Special Juice Mix

*200 ml fresh carrot juice*
*150 ml fresh celery juice*
*50 ml fresh beetroot juice*

Juice the vegetables and then strain the juice through muslin to make it pulp free. Store excess juice in the refrigerator. For best digestion, sip slowly.

# Ant Bite

*See Insect Bite Itch, Stings and Bites.*

# Antibiotics

Garlic, grapes, nasturtiums, radish and thyme are all natural antibiotics. During times of infection any or all of them can be included in your diet. However, make it a habit to include them permanently as a preventive measure.

Most of the essential oils are antibiotics and very strong bactericides.

Garlic, without doubt one of Mother Nature's best antibiotics, can be eaten as a vegetable, or as a soup (absolutely delicious and an excellent way to help combat the miseries of colds and flu), or you can buy odourless garlic tablets from health food stores. I make my own 'tablets' by slicing cloves into pill-sized portions, then simply popping a piece or two down my throat a couple of times a day. To combat the smell I chew on a sprig of fresh parsley afterwards. Mind you, if you decide to overdose yourself on a fresh garlic pill (which will do you no harm), the parsley may take care of the breath odour, but the odour that will exude from the pores of your skin may offend others.

*See also Garlic.*

# Antiseptic

A few drops of lavender or tea-tree oil in a cup of warm water makes an all-purpose antiseptic for cuts, scratches and abrasions. Apply with clean lint or cotton wool.

Alternatively, blend equal parts of eucalyptus oil and aloe vera juice and store in an amber-coloured glass bottle until needed. Best used for grazes and scratches. Keep no longer than 2 months.

The juice extracted from the fresh flowers of the echinacea plant is a natural antiseptic which can be used externally to treat bacterial infections and vaginal thrush.

## ANTISEPTIC AIR-SPRAY

This antiseptic spray has natural antifungal and antibacterial properties, and can be used in the bathroom, or to freshen a sickroom, or anywhere else an antiseptic spray is needed.

*25 drops lavender essential oil*
*10 drops lemon essential oil*
*5 drops eucalyptus essential oil*
*5 ml methylated spirits*
*500 ml distilled water*

Dissolve the essential oils in the methylated spirits and add this to a pump-spray bottle that contains the distilled water. Shake well to mix, and use on a fine mist spray as required.

*See also Echinacea, Tea-Tree Oil, Thyme.*

# Anxiety

*See Bathing, Chamomile (Chamomile Tea), Insomnia, Massage, Revitalisation, Sleep, Stress and Tension, Tonics.*

# Appetite Stimulants

Caraway tea drunk ½ hour before a meal, or whenever desired, is a powerful, natural appetite stimulant. Infuse 1 teaspoon of crushed, dried seeds in a cup of hot water (use a ceramic cup) for 5 minutes. Strain into another cup, reheat if required, and sweeten with honey to taste.

Another excellent appetite stimulant is horehound tea, especially when you are recovering from a cold or flu. Drink 1 cup of horehound tea 3 times a day.

# Aromatic Shower

Taking a warm shower after a workout is one of the best things you can do. It will not only make you feel good — all those negative ions you will be inhaling are extremely beneficial — but it will also help eliminate the lactic acid that causes your muscles to ache. However, showering with just soap and water will not provide the deep cleaning that your body requires. Using essential oils when you shower will help eliminate waste products from your body, thus preventing sore and aching muscles.

Before taking a shower, rub your body with a clean flannel to which you have added 3 drops each of rosemary, lemon and eucalyptus essential oil. Rub it all over yourself and then shower in the normal way.

After showering, massage your muscles with a relaxant body oil. To make your body oil, dissolve 6 drops of either lavender or rosemary essential oil in 20 ml of almond oil. Pour a little of the oil blend into the palm of your hand and massage it thoroughly into your legs and arms, using upward, circular movements towards your heart. Finish off by massaging your stomach and shoulder muscles.

An aromatic shower is a great way to start the day. Rub your entire body with a little body oil, made as previously, containing stimulating essences such as tangerine or lemon essential oil, diluted half-and-half with water. Plug the shower drain and, while showering, sprinkle in more of the aromatic oil as the water collects. Your feet will benefit from the fragrant soak, while the ascending aroma will make you feel alive and ready to take on the world.

*See also Muscular Aches and Pains.*

# Arthritis

Arthritic joints are very painful, and they are often stubborn in responding to treatment. It is important to maintain a simple diet and avoid salt, sugar, tea, margarine, nuts, vinegar, soft drinks, acidic fruits, dairy products (including ice-cream), red meat and wheat products. Fruit juice can be drunk, but only sparingly, and should be taken by the spoonful so that it will assimilate with saliva.

Include the following in your diet: oats, celery, parsley, mustard, fresh young nettles, white fish and poultry, lots of raw vegetables and salads, including plenty of cabbage (diced, sliced, cooked or boiled), and feverfew. This is an anti-inflammatory herb. Eat 3 fresh young leaves a day in a sandwich or take it in capsules (available from health food stores) or as a tea. Replace refined flour with either oats or bran.

Increase your vitamin and mineral intake, concentrating on additional calcium, vitamins C, B and D, and zinc. You should also drink 1 glass of carrot juice a day (or a combination of equal parts of fresh carrot and celery juice) and plenty of water.

Other inflammatory and soothing herbs are chamomile and meadowsweet; the latter is helpful with pain and inflammation in the joints. Take either herb as a tea 3–4 times a day.

Painful joints can be relieved by garlic ointment or Spirit of Balm being massaged into the affected area (*see Garlic Ointment, Spirit of Balm*). Rosemary essential oil also makes an excellent rub for inflamed and painful joints, and has a natural hyperaemic effect (increases local blood circulation). Dilute 5 ml of the essential oil with 50 ml of olive oil and store in an airtight, amber-coloured glass bottle away from direct sunlight or heat. Use whenever necessary.

*See also Alfalfa, Feverfew, Jojoba, Potassium, Rosemary, Salt.*

# Asthma

Asthma requires expert treatment and advice from your health practitioner. However, the problem can be aided by including the following in your diet — apples, carrots, figs, garlic, green peppers, horseradish, lemons, onions, oranges and raisins. A small glass of equal parts of fresh carrot juice and celery juice daily is also helpful.

To ease tightness and a chesty cough, fill a bottle of honey with honeysuckle flowers, ensuring that each is coated with honey, and take 2–3 spoonfuls of the mixture every day.

Herbal teas that are known to help:

▶ A cup of parsley tea each night before going to bed.
▶ A cup of fennel tea before bed for adults (½ cup for children). To make fennel tea, put 2 teaspoons of dried, crushed seed in 2 cups of milk, heat to just below boiling point, then simmer for 10 minutes. Make sure it doesn't boil over.
▶ Oregano or marjoram tea is also helpful when drunk during the day. Drink a small glass of the tea after meals.

*See Herbal Teas for preparation directions.*

*See also Allergies, Hay Fever, Medicinal Oils, Nasal Congestion, Oregano.*

# Astragalus

This popular Chinese energy tonic has recently become known to Western medicine through clinical studies into its properties as an immune strengthener. Astragalus (*Astragalus membranaceus*) stimulates white blood cell activity and increases the production of interferon, both vital components for a healthy immune system. It is available as a liquid extract from most natural therapists.

# Athlete's Foot

This is characterised by soft, peeling skin between the toes, leaving your feet clammy and quite often smelly. It is caused by a fungal infection which thrives where the acid balance of the skin has become too alkaline.

Athlete's foot is very infectious, so do not walk around barefoot where other people are likely to tread, or allow sharing of thongs, sandals or towels, or use the same bath mat. After drying between your toes, wash your towel in hot water and soap, with a few drops of lavender oil added. Don't use the towel on other parts of your body, as tinea can easily spread, especially to the groin area.

Treat with applications of cider vinegar over the affected area, or apply a fungicide made by dissolving 1 part tea-tree oil in 10 parts water.

Soak your feet in warm water to which has been added 6–10 drops of tea-tree or lavender oil. After washing and drying your feet, dust between your toes with powdered arrowroot.

For persistent cases, paint the affected area with neat tea-tree oil and place a cotton wool ball, moistened with several drops of oil, in your shoes at night.

Even when the fungus looks as though it has cleared, continue the treatment for a few more days, as this complaint is very persistent. You should also liberally sprinkle the floor tiles of your bathroom with neat lavender oil — its natural antiseptic and disinfect properties will kill the fungus.

## SPECIAL FUNGAL FOOTBATH

An ideal footbath for persistent fungal conditions, such as tinea.

*30 g dried soapwort root*
*3 tablespoons dried chamomile*
*3 litres water*

In an enamel or stainless steel pan bring the soapwort to the boil in 1 litre of water. Cover and simmer for 25 minutes. Remove from heat, and pour the herb and water liquid into a foot basin. Add the chamomile and 2 litres of boiling water. Cover and steep for 30 minutes. Strain, reheat and pour back into the basin.
Soak your feet for 15 minutes, then rinse your feet in a basin of cold water to which have been added 2 tablespoons of cider vinegar. Then dry your feet very thoroughly with a towel, which must be kept for your use only. Boil the towel after use.
Dust between your toes with powdered arrowroot when they are thoroughly dried.

*See also Aloe Vera, Feet, Fungal Problems, Thyme.*

# B

## Babies

We all know how miserable and unpleasant it is to feel ill. But it must be twice as bad for toddlers and young children who quite often may not understand what is happening to them.

There are a number of natural solutions that will enable you to deal with simple everyday situations. However, these remedies are suggestions only. If you are unsure of your child's problem or it is an acute situation, contact your health practitioner.

### COLIC

Colic is a very common problem with young ones and causes a great deal of discomfort. An old-fashioned remedy to relieve gas and flatulence in windy babies is to give them 1 teaspoon of dill water as needed. You can purchase dill water from chemists.

### CRADLE CAP

This is another source of discomfort for young ones. You can make a soothing lotion by bringing ⅓ cup of dried chamomile flowers almost to the boil in 150 ml of olive oil. Remove from heat, allow to cool, then strain through sterile muslin cloth into an airtight, sterilised glass bottle. Use as needed by rubbing the chamomile oil gently into the scalp, then washing the scalp off with warm soapy water.

Another solution is to apply aloe vera lotion to the scalp and brush gently. Aloe vera can be purchased as a stabilised lotion from most health food shops.

## NAPPY RASH

To soothe the irritation of nappy rash, apply garlic oil to the affected area. To make the oil, chop up 6 garlic cloves and add them and 500 ml of sunflower oil to a glass jar. Seal tightly, leave to stand for 10 days, then strain and store in an airtight glass bottle.

Alternatively, bathe the affected area with Chamomile Nappy Wash whenever the nappy is changed. Put 1 cup each of dried chamomile flowers and dried elder flowers into a ceramic bowl, add sufficient boiling water to cover by about 2 cm, then cover the bowl and leave it to infuse overnight. Strain through clean muslin cloth and store in a sterilised, airtight bottle in the refrigerator. The mixture will not keep any longer than 7 days. If it begins to smell off any earlier, discard it and make a fresh batch.

## TEETHING

For a teething baby, rub aloe vera gel on the gums or steep 1 or 2 chamomile tea bags (available from health food shops) in 1 cup of hot water. Add a little powdered ginger to taste. Strain and give 1 teaspoon frequently.

If the infant won't settle, add a few drops of chamomile tea to its milk bottle. This will also soothe cramp or colic in the bowels.

*See also Chamomile.*

# Bad Breath

Bad breath is usually a result of congestion in the colon. Add 2 drops of peppermint oil to 1 cup of warm water, gargle for a few minutes then rinse out your mouth. Repeat as often as needed. You can also try chewing a fragrant cardamom pod or anise seeds 2–3 times a day.

The following 'Green Herbal Drink' is also excellent for bad breath, as well as being highly nutritious and cleansing. Make this fresh each day and drink morning and night.

### Green Herbal Drink

*250 g wild herbs (mixed or on their own): chickweed, fat hen, dandelion*
*2 tablespoons finely chopped parsley and/or watercress or celery*
*1 teaspoon cider vinegar*
*1 small carrot, chopped*
*250 g fruit (apple, peaches, pineapple or watermelon)*
*250 ml liquid to dilute (orange juice, pineapple juice or mineral water)*

Process all ingredients in a blender and drink immediately.

Include peas, potatoes, brown rice and barley in your diet.

*See also Oral Hygiene.*

# Bathing

Centuries ago, baths were rarely taken to actually cleanse the body; in combination with various herbs, they were used as a cure. Today, a bath can still be used to restore your body, to soothe tired muscles and refresh your mind in the same way a good night's sleep can.

The addition of rosemary essential oil will stimulate your circulation and soften your skin; lavender will also soften your skin, as well as providing unique disinfecting properties. Chamomile oil in your bathwater works in the same way as it does when its flowers are drunk as a herbal tea. It calms your nerves and relaxes your body in preparation for a sound, natural sleep.

For a real get-up-and-go bath that will make you feel invigorated and alive, add peppermint or lemon essential oil to the water. And to just relax and let the world drift on by, add 2 drops each of chamomile and rose essential oil and 6 drops of lavender essential oil.

Before adding your essential oils the bathwater, dissolve them in about 20 ml of cider vinegar. Approximately 6–10 drops of your chosen oil will be sufficient. The addition of the cider vinegar will help combat dryness of the skin by restoring its acid balance.

## PREPARATIONS FOR SPECIAL PURPOSES:

The following herbal bath suggestions should all be added to the bath in a bath bag, and can be varied to suit your requirements.

### A Refreshing Bath

*Spearmint, lavender, lemon verbena, salad burnet*

### To Ease Tired and Aching Muscles

*Rosemary, bay leaf, honeysuckle, hyssop, angelica, lovage, chamomile*

### To Invigorate and Rejuvenate

*Rosemary, lovage, lavender, nettle, valerian, peppermint, comfrey*

### To Relax, Soothe, Calm and Promote Sleep

*Chamomile, lovage, lime flowers, pennyroyal, rosemary, yarrow*

### To Comfort Tired and Frazzled Nerves

*Pennyroyal, rosemary, bay leaf, chamomile, lime flowers, valerian*

### To Soothe Sore Skin

*Comfrey, marigold (Calendula), woodruff, violets, lady's mantle, marshmallow, chamomile, elder flowers*

For a relaxing bath, cook some fine oatmeal until soft, then transfer the solids and all the soothing liquids to a muslin bag. Hang the bag in the bathwater so that the liquid can work its soothing magic.

## BATH BAG

To make a bath bag, take a 20 cm square of muslin, place the herbs in the centre, draw up the sides and tie with a piece of ribbon. For maximum effect, hang the bag from the tap so that the hot water gushes through it. Rub the bag briskly over your body like a sponge, then lie back and relax in the fragrant water.

# DRY BATHING

*See Dry Bathing.*

## MOISTURISING BATH

Skin suffers from the harshness of winter, the cold winds leaving it dry and rough. All those clothes that we pile on to keep warm do nothing for our skin either; once they are peeled off, a grey pallor, complete with rough, cracked areas, is often revealed.

The simplest way to moisturise your body while bathing is to add a few drops of almond oil to the water. Your skin will soon be looking and feeling supple again.

## NOURISHING BATH OIL

Dilute 40 drops of rose oil and 10 drops of lavender oil in 10 ml of avocado oil, 10 ml of wheat germ oil and 30 ml of almond oil. Put this oil blend in a dark-coloured, airtight bottle and shake well until thoroughly mixed.

Add 1 teaspoon of this mixture to your bathwater to nourish, soften and moisturise your skin.

## SODA BATH

Soda baths are marvellous for soothing itching skin, and for relieving vaginitis.

To prepare a bath, add ½ cup of bicarbonate of soda to the bathwater. Swish it around until it dissolves, then lie back and relax.

## VINEGAR BATH

This special addition to your bath will help combat dry skin by restoring its acid balance.

Combine 10 ml of cider vinegar and 90 ml of distilled water in a suitable bottle, seal, and shake until well blended.

Brush your skin with the vinegar solution using a loofah, as you would for dry bathing (*see Dry Bathing*). This will help loosen dead skin cells and improve circulation. Rinse off any residue in a warm bath.

---

*See also Aromatic Shower, Aching Joints and Muscles, Muscular Aches and Pains.*

# Bee Stings

---

*See Insect Bite Itch, Stings and Bites.*

# Bilberry

Commonly know as an eye herb, bilberry (*Vaccinium myrtillus*) has a reputation for helping to strengthen eyesight, and for preventing and treating eye disorders such as macular degeneration, night blindness and cataracts. Flavonoid compounds, the active ingredients in bilberry, are known to support biochemical reactions and strengthen the capillaries in the eye that are responsible for eyesight.

Bilberry is available in tablet or capsule form from health food stores and some chemists. It is also available combined with other beneficial eye herbs, as a supplement.

---

*See also Eyes.*

# Black Eye

Soothe with a paste of bicarbonate of soda and a cold cloth.

# Blackheads

*See Acne.*

# Blisters

Apply 1 drop of lavender essential oil to the affected spot, patting it in thoroughly but carefully.

## BLISTERS FROM BURNS AND SCALDS

Under no circumstances pierce the blister. Apply 1 drop of lavender essential oil to the blister, and then hold an ice cube on it for 10 minutes. Cover with a lavender compress, and repeat the procedure up to 3 times a day.

To make a lavender compress, add 10 drops of essential oil to 100 ml of water. Soak a piece of cloth in the liquid, then remove it and squeeze it gently until it stops dripping. Apply it to the affected area and cover with plastic wrap.

*See also Feet, Geranium, Prickly Heat.*

# Blood Pressure

It is important to ensure that you include plenty of fresh green salad vegetables in your daily diet.

## HIGH BLOOD PRESSURE

Include in your diet broccoli, barley, carrots, cauliflower, celery, chives, cucumbers, endive, garlic, onions, oranges, parsley, peaches, pears, peppers (capsicum), pineapples, spinach, squash, strawberries, tomatoes, yarrow tea and cayenne pepper.

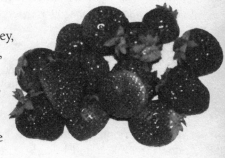

## LOW BLOOD PRESSURE

Your diet should include nuts (such as walnuts, Brazil nuts and pecan nuts), currants, dates, figs, garlic, leeks, peas, pumpkin, pumpkin seeds, raisins, soya beans, sweet potato and young dandelion greens (slightly steamed or chopped and added to a salad).

**Warning:** *Blood pressure is a serious condition and should not be treated without first consulting with your health practitioner.*

*See also Exercise, Nutrition (Refined Sugar), Yarrow.*

# Body Odour

Include the herbs parsley, sage and celery in your diet.

One or 2 drops of essential oil of lavender dabbed under your arms and on other areas will reduce body odour for about 6 hours in warm climates, and longer where it is cold. If you mix the oil with a little sorbolene it will last even longer.

You can make your own deodorant by dissolving lavender oil, a drop at a time, in 10 ml of cider vinegar until the vinegar smells like lavender. Then add the mixture to 250 ml of distilled water. Shake well to mix, then store in an airtight glass bottle. Dab under arms and other areas as needed.

# Borage

Borage is one of the oldest known herbs used by the human race. Both the flowers and the leaves have a therapeutic action.

Fresh young leaves are an ideal addition to salads. When taken as a tea, borage exerts a beneficial influence on the liver, uterus, chest, stomach and bowels. The tea can also be used to stimulate the adrenal glands and as a purifier for other body systems. Mixed with basil it will assist both the bladder and kidneys. In the seventeenth century, a decoction of borage leaves, bran and barley was recommended as an additive to bathwater to cleanse and soften the skin. Leaves applied as a compress to the veins of the legs will relieve congestion and prevent varicose veins.

The flowers, which can be picked and eaten straight from the plant, are very tasty and rich in both nectar and silicic acid; the latter aids the healthy growth of hair and nails, and the lining of the mucous membranes.

Purchase the seeds or plant from a nursery or specialist herb nursery. Once planted in the garden it will freely reseed every year.

## BORAGE OINTMENT

Use this ointment for itchy and bleeding haemorrhoids.

*2 tablespoons dried borage leaves or 1 handful fresh leaves*
*100 ml glycerine*

Put all the ingredients in a small ceramic bowl and place this in a pan of boiling water. Simmer over low heat for 30 minutes. Remove, strain, and discard the herbs. Store in a sterilised, airtight glass bottle and use as needed.

# Breast Care

Although the shape and size of breasts differ from woman to woman and are governed by many factors, such as age, obesity and weight reduction, it is still important to tone and firm the pectoral muscles and to keep the skin of the breast smooth and healthy. Essential oils are helpful here, and should be used after a bath or shower, when the skin is still warm and slightly moist. Massage with the fingers and palms, using small circular movements inwards from the outer sides of each breast, and then upwards from below each breast. Maintain strong firm strokes, pressing upwards over the nipples and up to just under the chin.

Exercising, by imitating the breast stroke movement out of water, and by pushing against the hands when they are placed at chin level with your elbows stuck out either side, is beneficial. This will strengthen your pectoral muscles and improve breast tone by keeping the fibrous tissue supple.

### Breast Massage Oil

*30 ml grapeseed oil*
*12 drops lemon grass essential oil*
*3 drops sage essential oil*
*5 drops geranium essential oil*
*4 drops fennel essential oil*
*6 drops carrot oil*

Blend all oils thoroughly together and use immediately after a bath or shower. Store any excess oil in an airtight, amber-coloured glass bottle and use within 2 months. This treatment should be applied every day.

# Burns

Immediately apply a cloth soaked in ice water, keeping the cloth wet and cold until the pain leaves. As an emergency dressing, apply the inside of a banana skin or the inner side of a piece of potato peel, holding it in place with a loosely bound bandage.

Apply the inner, jelly-like substance of an aloe vera leaf (*Aloe barbadensis* — medicinal aloe) to the painful area. Aloe vera soothes the burn, immediately takes away the pain, and promotes quick healing that doesn't leave a scar. The oil quickly penetrates the skin, carrying nutrients deep into the epidermis where they are needed; it is an excellent remedy for both heat and acid burns.

For minor household burns caused by touching a hot iron or grasping an overheated saucepan handle, gently pat lavender oil onto the affected area.

**Warning:** *Serious burns, especially those to young children or to a large part of the body, require immediate emergency medical attention.*

## ALOE VERA LOTION

For burns, broken skin, scratches and wounds.

*10 ml glycerine*
*12 ml olive oil*
*12 ml wheat germ oil*
*6 drops calendula oil*
*20 ml aloe vera juice*
*45 ml rosewater*

Add all the ingredients to an amber-coloured glass bottle, seal tightly and shake well. Shake well again before using.

---

*See also Honeysuckle (Honeysuckle Ointment), Sunburn.*

# Burping

Burping or belching is caused by eating too quickly and drinking too much fluid with your meals. Try eating slowly and reducing your fluid intake during meals. A cup of peppermint tea after your meal will help give relief, as will a garlic or vitamin tablet soaked in peppermint oil.

# Butter and Margarine

Butter and margarine possess a number of similar properties when related to the human diet. Their purpose is to make bread more appealing and appetising, and there is no doubt that bread is popular today because of these two spreads. The difference between butter and margarine is that margarine is not a milk product.

Cheaper margarines were once manufactured from whale blubber, and were even higher in fatty acids than butter. Today the product is manufactured from polyunsaturated vegetable oils. Unfortunately, a great deal of the polyunsaturated advantage is lost during the margarine's processing. But at least this product is derived from vegetable oils and is cholesterol free.

You can easily substitute natural, cold-pressed vegetable oils for butter or margarine in cooking. In fact, coconut oil is a perfect substitute; it is pure, more easily digested, and can be used as an anti-stick oil for wiping over the surface of baking pans and the like.

If you would like to try a different spread on your bread, there are dairy-free butter substitutes made from soya flour and oil or yeast, olive oil and kelp (*see Dietary Substitutes*).

# C

## Calcium

The body contains more calcium than any other mineral, and it is calcium that ensures healthy bones and teeth and the proper processing of all vitamins in the food we consume. It stimulates enzyme activity and is important for a healthy heart and for the nerves associated with the heart.

Weight-bearing exercise, such as walking, cycling and swimming, and vitamin D are essential to stimulate calcium's absorption into the body. However, high-protein diets, high salt intake and caffeine, nicotine and alcohol will all destroy calcium.

Natural food sources are: alfalfa, almonds, Brazil nuts, broccoli, dandelion greens, eggs, fish and oysters, garlic, leafy green vegetables, milk and milk products, molasses, nettle (young leaves), parsley, prawns, salmon, sardines, sesame seeds, skim milk, soya beans, tofu, sunflower seeds, yogurt, watercress and wheat germ.

## Calendula

Calendula (*Calendula officinalis*), made into a tincture or ointment, is by far one of the finest remedies for scratches, grazes, cuts and all open wounds. The oil is a natural antiseptic, and as soon as it is applied the healing process commences. Calendula ointment will also act as a soothing balm for insect bites.

An infusion of the petals in a footbath will soothe aching feet, and the essential oil will remove soreness when it is rubbed into them.

The dried herb is available from health food stores. Calendula products, such as ointments, creams and tinctures, are available from health food stores, chemists and supermarkets that have a health products section.

---

*See also Cuts and Grazes, Stings and Bites.*

# Calluses and Corns

Calluses and corns are usually a result of neglecting your feet. One of the best treatments for these conditions is Golden Seal ointment, available from herbalists, specialty herbal suppliers and some health food stores. It has a softening, soothing and normalising action on callused skin, corns and bunions.

Massage the ointment thoroughly into the hardened area until it is completely absorbed, and as often as necessary until the problem is alleviated.

Other remedies which will soften calluses and corns are:

▶ Soak your feet in a footbath of strong chamomile tea. Prepare the tea by infusing 2 tablespoons of dried herb per litre of hot water. Infuse overnight, strain the chamomile through clean muslin cloth, and reheat the liquid before soaking your feet.
▶ Chop up a piece of comfrey leaf and squeeze out as much of the juice as possible. Apply the juice to the affected spot each night and cover with a gauze bandage.
▶ Rub the corn every night with a crushed garlic clove, or put a sliver of garlic on the corn and hold it on with sticking plaster.
▶ Apply freshly crushed marigold (calendula) leaves to the corn morning and night.

# Catarrh

My grandmother would swear by her leek and ginger soup for the relief of catarrh associated with colds and flu.

## LEEK AND GINGER SOUP

Trim, rinse and slice 3 leeks and grate sufficient fresh ginger to make 1 tablespoon. Gently heat 1 tablespoon of olive oil in a large pan and sauté the leeks for about 10 minutes, without browning them. Add the grated ginger and 1 litre of water. Cover, bring to the boil, and allow to simmer for 20 minutes, until the leeks are tender. Season to taste with fresh parsley and thyme.

*See also Colds.*

# Chamomile

Almost everyone is familiar with the herb chamomile and its yellow and white daisy-like flowers that are used to make the popular tea. But are you aware that it is one of the safest and gentlest of all the herbs?

The ancient Egyptians dedicated chamomile to the sun, and the tea has been known and respected for centuries for its soothing and calming qualities; German chamomile (*Matricaria recutica*) is the most effective. In Europe many people drink a cup of this herbal tea as their customary nightcap, to relax them before going to bed.

Chamomile tea has a light, apple-like taste and is rich in calcium. It is a time-honoured remedy for gastro-intestinal disorders, menstrual pain, nerves, and migraine headaches. A cup of chamomile tea at night is said to induce sound natural sleep and calm an overactive brain. It is an ideal drink at study time or when you are under stress, and students and tired business people will benefit from a cup of chamomile tea at the end of every day.

A few drops added occasionally to a baby's milk bottle will help calm and settle a restless infant; it will also soothe cramp or colic in the bowels when used as gripe water. To make Infant's Gripe Water, put 1 teaspoon of dried chamomile in an enamel or stainless steel pan, add 300 ml of boiling water and simmer for 5 minutes. Remove from heat, allow to cool, strain, add honey and use tepid in baby's bottle.

A strong brew of the tea can be poured into an evening bath to help relax and soothe tired muscles. It can also be used as a compress or eye bath for the treatment of red, inflamed eyes. Just add the cold tea to an eyeglass and bathe the eyes.

Because of its low toxicity, chamomile is especially suitable for children. It will soothe skin disorders such as acne, burns, stings and rashes, and is excellent for conjunctivitis, infant's teething problems, rheumatism and neuralgia. To ease rheumatism and other aches and pains, massage the affected spot with a blend of 25 ml of soya oil and 2 drops each of chamomile and rosemary oil.

To soothe skin irritations, make a lotion by combining 5 tablespoons of olive oil, 10 drops of chamomile oil and 5 drops of Borneo camphor, and dab it onto the skin with a piece of cotton wool.

Conjunctivitis can be treated by mixing 1 drop of chamomile oil with 1 teaspoon of witch hazel, and blending this solution with 30 ml of rosewater. Let it stand for 8 hours, strain through coffee filter paper, and use with a compress on the eyelids. Be sure to keep your eyes closed.

## CHAMOMILE SOAP

A good herbal soap exerts its effects on the outer layer of the skin — the so-called horny or epithelial layer — making it smooth and soft. Chamomile soap is both smoothing and healing to the skin, and is suitable for all skin types, including skin affected by acne and other similar problems. It is also ideal for men to use, as it will soothe facial skin that suffers from the trauma of daily shaving.

To make your soap, first put 5 tablespoons of dried chamomile in a ceramic bowl and add 300 ml of boiling water. Cover the bowl with a plate, steep for 12 hours, then strain through muslin or cheesecloth, squeezing all liquid from the herbs, and add to the following recipe.

Melt 350 g of grated, pure white soap in an enamel pan over a low heat with just enough of the chamomile infusion to form a soft paste (use a potato masher to help dissolve the soap). Add the remaining infusion and stir continuously until thoroughly blended. Remove the mixture from the heat source and pour it into suitable moulds. Leave the soap to harden before removing it from the moulds. Your soap is ready to use as soon as it has set.

Moulds for the soap mixture can be small, shallow cardboard boxes, clean milk cartons or anything suitable. You can increase the quantity of the recipe proportionately to make more soap.

*See also Acne, Babies, Conjunctivitis, Eyes, Hair, Insomnia, Muscular Aches and Pains, Neuralgia, Rashes, Rheumatism, Skin Care, Skin Irritations, Sleep.*

# Chapped Lips

Apply the following lip balm whenever required to keep your lips moist and supple, and to prevent them chapping or splitting.

Melt 15 g of beeswax in a double pan over a medium heat. When completely liquid, stir in 50 ml of almond oil, 10 ml of wheat germ oil, 5 ml of jojoba oil and 40 ml of distilled water and mix until well blended. Remove from heat and pour into a ceramic bowl. Add 6 drops of friar's balsam and 5 drops each of chamomile and rose essential oil. Beat until cool and creamy. Store in a sterilised glass jar.

*See also Jojoba, Skin (Protection).*

# Chilblains

Mix 1 tablespoon each of honey and glycerine, 1 teaspoon of rosewater, the white of an egg, and sufficient flour to make a paste. Wash the affected area with warm water, then dry it and spread on the paste. Cover with a piece of sterile linen or cotton bandage.

A footbath of potato-peel water is also reputed to be a remedy for chilblains. Another remedy is to mash up the inside of a baked potato, mix it with a little sunflower oil, and apply it warm to the affected spot.

For broken chilblains, make a very strong infusion of calendula petals and comfrey leaves. Cool to body temperature, strain out the herbs, and soak your feet in the infusion until it is no longer warm. Then apply the strained herb pulp as a poultice, leaving it on as long as possible. Repeat the procedure as necessary.

Include the following in your diet: fresh young dandelion greens, cayenne, ginger (as a condiment), figs and guavas.

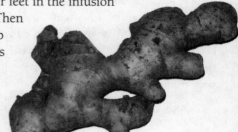

# Chilli

A herb found in most homes, chilli (*Capsicum* spp.) is known to have a beneficial effect on the entire digestive system and the circulatory system, increasing blood flow, metabolism and appetite. It is mildly antibacterial and makes an excellent gargle for sore throats and laryngitis, especially when combined with herbs such as thyme and lavender. When used in conjunction with other herbs it acts as a catalyst, accentuating their action by increasing their power and speeding up the beneficial effect.

Chilli is available from fruit and vegetable shops, and the plants and seeds are available from most nurseries and from the garden section of large variety stores.

**Warning:** *Never take medicinal amounts of this herb when you are pregnant or breastfeeding, and never take large medicinal doses unless under medical supervision; it can lead to liver damage.*

# Cholesterol

*See Eating for Health and Energy (Lecithin, Oats, Soluble Fibre), Eggs, Exercise, Garlic, Iron, Vitamin F, Zinc.*

# Chlorine

Chlorine combines with natural sodium to act as a body cleanser. Because large quantities of this mineral exist as chlorides in most foods, we don't need to choose specific food groups to obtain it. However, using common salt is not the appropriate way to absorb chlorine into the body. The same applies to sodium.

Some natural food sources of chlorine are: asparagus, avocados, bananas, chives, Brussels sprouts, dandelion greens, eggplants, figs, guavas, mangoes, peaches, pineapples, raisins, sunflower seeds, sweet potato and watermelon.

# Circulation

To improve circulation and sweeten your blood, include plenty of fresh garden peas in your diet.

Take 1 cup of rosehip tea 3 times a day to help reduce circulatory problems. An infusion of the herb rosemary added to your bathwater will also stimulate your circulation.

# Cod Liver Oil

Cod liver oil contains the essential fatty acids Eicosapentaenoic acid and Docosahexaenoic acid (both of which are Omega 3 fatty acids). They support healthy cholesterol levels as part of a low-fat diet, and are an excellent source of vitamins A, D and K.

Vitamins A and D support healthy joints, bones, skin, hair and teeth, as well as helping to maintain your body's natural defences and contributing to healthy eyes and vision; vitamin K is essential for the blood's clotting action. Cod liver oil should be avoided by pregnant women, asthmatics, diabetics and people taking anticoagulant drugs. It can also cause nausea, so it is best taken with meals.

Cod liver oil is available as a supplement from health food stores, chemists and the health food section of supermarkets.

# Coffee Substitute

Most people have felt the adverse effects of caffeine — from drinking too much coffee — and know that a healthier alternative is to substitute it by drinking herbal tea. But how many people realise that there are natural replacements to coffee? These natural replacements are not only caffeine free; they also provide a refreshing taste alternative.

Dandelion coffee substitute, made from the dried, roasted and ground roots of this humble weed, is readily available from health food stores and some supermarkets. This healthy alternative is a virtual storehouse of vitamins, minerals, enzymes, proteins and other valuable elements, making it a wholesome plant food. Taken on a regular basis it acts as a general tonic.

If you prefer to make your own dandelion coffee substitute, gather fresh roots in autumn from an area that has not been affected by herbicide or insecticide spraying (these elements can become even more harmful after heating). Cut the roots into rings about 2 cm thick and dry them in the sun on drying trays (muslin cloth stretched over a timber frame will suffice). Do not leave them out overnight where they will attract moisture.

Once completely dry, roast the pieces of root in a hot oven (200°C) for 20 minutes. Reduce the roasted root to granules in a coffee bean grinder or blender, and store in an airtight jar. Use in the same way as instant coffee.

Other natural alternatives to coffee are chicory, sunflower seeds and wattle seeds. Chicory coffee substitute is available in health food stores and supermarkets. This perennial herb is a lovely plant to have growing in the garden, with tall blue stalks of flowers over most of the summer. Its roots can be dug at any time — they are at their sweetest in autumn — and turned into a homemade caffeine-free beverage.

Chicory coffee is made the same way as dandelion coffee. Use 1 dessertspoonful of the ground root to 1 cup of boiling water.

To make sunflower seed coffee, roast the unhulled seeds in a slow oven (150°C) until they are quite brittle, then grind them finely in a blender or other food processor. Use 2 dessertspoons of ground seed to 1 cup of boiling water.

Wattle seeds also make a coffee with an interesting taste. However, some wattles' seeds are bitter — taste them first. If they taste sweet, dry them, grind them up and use them as you would use instant coffee.

The next time you feel like a cuppa, try one of the caffeine-free alternatives! You will be pleasantly surprised.

# Colds

Immediate treatment of colds and flu will raise your immunity levels as well as alleviate your symptoms. Garlic in your daily diet will help build a natural resistance to colds and also help your auto-immune system cope with bacterial infection. It contains vitamins A, B and C, and copper, sulphur, manganese, iron and calcium, and because its oil is composed of sulphides and disulphides, it deactivates undesirable virulent micro-organisms in your body without harming the helpful organisms.

However, you must be mindful of the fact that no matter how you take fresh garlic, after a while your body fragrance will be astounding. If others around you find this offensive, try odourless garlic tablets, which are available from health food stores.

Your diet should also include plenty of vitamin C (500–1000 mg a day), carrots, spinach, oranges, grapefruit, guavas, horseradish (freshly grated on bread), onions, chives, green peppers, cabbage, Brussels sprouts, tomatoes and turnips.

## FIRST SIGN OF A COLD

At the first sign of a cold, add 1 drop of eucalyptus or tea-tree oil to a glass of warm water and gargle.

## BUILDING UP IMMUNITY

To help build up your body's immunity or ease the symptoms of colds and flu, drink 1 cupful of garlic brew 3 times a day.

*See Garlic (Garlic Cold Cure).*

## HERBAL TEA FOR COLDS

Combine equal parts peppermint, elder flower and yarrow. Infuse 1 teaspoon of the dried herb mixture in 1 cup of boiling water for 10 minutes. Strain, reheat, sweeten with honey and drink as hot as possible 3–4 times a day, including before going to bed.

Peppermint is rich in volatile oils, including menthol, which help relieve head and chest congestion. Taken on its own, peppermint tea is very beneficial in reducing fever; its effect is increased when it is combined with yarrow flowers. Peppermint also helps to reduce nausea and acts as a soothing sedative to induce relaxation and sleep.

Elder flowers are rich in the mineral salt potassium chloride, which is vital for dealing with the second-stage congestion of colds, flu and fevers. They have a relaxing and calming effect, help purify the blood, and induce perspiration.

Yarrow is useful for treating mild fevers, as it produces perspiration and opens the pores of the skin. (Free perspiration encourages the elimination of toxins and waste products from the body. Poor elimination of perspiration is one of the primary factors in the development of colds, fevers and flu.) This herb also contains the mineral salt iron phosphate, which is especially effective in treating infectious colds and fevers.

To accentuate the action of this herbal tea and speed up its beneficial effects, add a pinch of cayenne pepper; it is both stimulating and warming and acts as a catalyst.

## SHIVERY COLD

A clove of garlic taken 3 times a day, with meals, will help alleviate symptoms, and is even more effective when taken in conjunction with ½ teaspoon of horseradish powder in some warm water.

## FEVERISH COLD

Put the juice of ½ lemon into 1 cup of boiling water, add a peppermint tea bag and steep for 5 minutes, then sweeten with honey. Reheat if required. Drink 3–6 times a day.

## SORE THROAT

A sore throat can be eased by gargling with Sage tea or Rose Petal Throat Soother (below) as required. Honeysuckle syrup taken frequently by the teaspoonful will also give relief.

**Warning:** *Sage tea should be avoided during pregnancy, as it can bring on menstrual flow.*

Sucking on raspberries is an old-fashioned remedy for easing a swollen, sore throat. It can also help mouth ulcers.

### Rose Petal Throat Soother

*1 cup rose petals (fresh or dried)*
*200 g honey*

Put the ingredients into a bowl, then place the bowl in a shallow pan of boiling water and simmer for 10 minutes. Strain and store in a glass jar and seal tightly.
Either sip a teaspoonful or add to warm water and gargle.

### Dry and Mucus Throat

Gargle fennel tea as needed.

## SPECIAL BATH FOR COLDS

Close all windows and the bathroom door for maximum effect. Run the bathwater as hot as you can stand it, and when the bath is almost full add 2 drops each of pine, eucalyptus and cypress essential oil. Swish the water around to ensure that the oils are thoroughly blended.

Sit with your knees up and your head between them so that you can fully inhale the restorative vapours. As the water cools, slosh it all over your body.

If you feel really ill, or nauseated, or running a fever, do not take a full bath; instead, run a shallow bath, sponge under your arms and around your genitals, and inhale until there is no more aromatic vapour.

Get out, vigorously dry yourself with a warm towel and then wrap yourself in another dry, warm towel for a few minutes. Finish off by massaging your entire body with the following oil: 2 drops of tea-tree oil and 3 drops of eucalyptus oil dissolved in 1 teaspoon of sunflower oil.

## CONGESTION

Use an inhalant to relieve all congestion, from the sinuses to the chest. Add a few drops of eucalyptus oil to a bowl of boiling water, place your face about 30 cm away from the bowl, and drape a towel over your head to form a tent. Do not let the steam escape, do not inhale steam for any longer than 10 minutes, and don't do it more than 3 times a day. (People with heart and blood pressure problems, asthma or other breathing difficulties, broken skin or visible, dilated red veins should avoid using steam inhalations, unless otherwise directed by their health practitioner.)

Eucalyptus oil penetrates right to the root of infection to exert its antiseptic action. It will also help laryngitis and other throat problems, as well as dry, aching or raw sinuses.

## PORTABLE INHALANT

Place a couple of drops of eucalyptus oil or 1 drop each of thyme, peppermint, eucalyptus and clove oil on a tissue. Carry the tissue with you, and inhale deeply from it whenever possible.

## OIL RUB

Before retiring, massage around your chest, neck and sinus area (forehead, nose and cheekbones) with the following oil blend: 1 drop of lemon oil, 2 drops of eucalyptus oil, 3 drops of rosemary oil and 1 teaspoon of almond oil.

## HERBAL CHEST RUB

To ease chest congestion, rub the following ointment liberally onto the skin around your upper chest and neck, just before going to bed.

*½ handful dried horseradish root*
*(or 1 tablespoon horseradish powder)*
*200 g petroleum jelly*

Reduce the horseradish root to a powder by rubbing it through a fine metal sieve or processing it in a blender. (Powdered horseradish is available from most health food stores.) Horseradish can burn sensitive skin, so do a patch test first.
Put the petroleum jelly into a small ceramic or glass bowl and place the bowl in a pan of boiling water. Stir the petroleum jelly until it has melted and then stir in the horseradish, making sure that it is well blended. Simmer the mixture for 20 minutes, then remove it from heat and store in a sterilised glass jar.

## INDUCING PERSPIRATION

Sprinkle cayenne pepper on your food and mix it with your herbal teas. It induces perspiration, which brings down fever and eliminates poisons and bacteria from your body.

# HEALING SOUP

*See Onion Soup, Garlic Soup.*

*See also Catarrh.*

## PROTECTING CHILDREN FROM WINTER COLDS

The front-line attack is to build up the body's resistance to infection. A wholefood diet that includes plenty of fresh fruit and vegetables and fresh herbs, including garlic, will help the body combat harmful bacteria and viruses. Rosehip tea, reputed to be high in vitamin C, can also be used to build resistance to colds and other infections.

## WHEN A COLD STRIKES A CHILD

Most colds will also respond to fruity treats. Add the juice of ½ lemon to 1 cup of boiling water and sweeten with honey. Take 3 times a day.

Essential oils can also be effective, and are very efficient at destroying harmful bacteria and viruses. Mix together 50 drops each of eucalyptus, tea-tree and lavender oil and store in an airtight, amber-coloured glass bottle. At bedtime, place a small bowl of boiling water, to which you have added 3 drops of the above blend of oils, under the bed or cot, but not directly under the child's head. The steam will rise, releasing the aroma into the room throughout the night. Do this again during the day.

If breathing is very difficult, place 2 drops of the oil blend on a cotton wool ball and place it under the edge of the child's pillow, or apply the drops to the pillow or pillowslip directly.

One drop of the oil blend can also be added to baby's bathwater. For children of 1–5 years, add 2 drops to the bath.

For older children, vaporising is also effective in relieving a stuffy or blocked-up nose. Moisten a small sponge with boiling water and add a few drops of the essential oil blend. Place the sponge in a dish in the child's room. Moisten it with boiling water twice a day, and refresh it with a few drops of the oil twice a week.

It must be remembered, however, that colds can be the forerunner of something more serious. So if the child has a temperature, is feverish, off food or crying or whingeing a lot, consult your health practitioner.

## NATURAL MEDICINE

The following natural medicine can be given to children by the tablespoonful twice a day to help build resistance or alleviate the miseries of a cold.

Slice 500 g of peeled onions into small rings. Put them in an enamel or stainless steel saucepan and add 2 litres of water, 80 g of honey, and 500 g of brown sugar. Simmer for 4 hours. Cool, strain through a fine sieve and bottle the liquid for future use.

*See also Echinacea, Garlic (Garlic Cold Cure), Horseradish,*
  *Lavender, Nasal Congestion.*

# Cold Sores

A good diet will help prevent cold sores. Include plenty of fresh fruit and vegetables, beans (pulses), chicken, fish and brewer's yeast. Avoid eating bread, oats, red meat, chocolate, sugar, coffee and hot spices, and spending unnecessary time in the sun.

To treat a cold sore, apply tea-tree oil as soon as it appears. Repeat the procedure 3–4 times a day for up to, but not more than, 5 days.

*See also Tea-Tree Oil.*

# Conjunctivitis

The discomfort of conjunctivitis can be eased by washing your eye with eyebright tea, which is available from most health food stores.

To make the tea, place 1 teaspoon of the dried herb in a ceramic cup and fill the cup with boiling water. Allow to cool, then strain, and wash the affected eye using an eyeglass. You can also soak a small cloth in the tea and use it as a compress on your eyelids.

*See also Chamomile.*

# Compresses

A therapeutic compress, using essential oils, can be used to treat many minor health problems. To make one, soak a piece of cotton gauze or a handkerchief in a bowl of hot water, to which the appropriate essential oil has been added (***see below***). Compresses work by drawing new blood and lymph to the affected area and absorbing the toxins. This method is therefore ideal for treating bruises, wounds, sprains, chest pains and skin problems.

To make your compress, add 10 drops of the appropriate essential oil to 100 ml of water (which can be either hot or cold, depending upon your need).

Soak the piece of cloth in the liquid, then remove it and gently squeeze it until it stops dripping. Apply the compress to the affected area and cover with plastic wrap. To increase the compress's ability to retain heat and thus be absorbed through the skin, wrap it with a pre-warmed towel, then place a blanket over the towel and the patient. The compress should be kept on the affected area for at least 2 hours.

Hot compresses can also be used to soothe old injuries, sprains, muscular aches and pains, neuralgia, painful periods and skin problems. A cold compress should be used to treat recent sprains, bruises or swellings and headaches. Cold compresses are far more effective if they are refrigerated first.

A number of common problems can be treated effectively with compresses made with the following essential oils:

▶ Bruises and bumps — *lavender, hyssop, calendula, rosemary or geranium.*

- Chilblains — *lavender, lemon, rosemary, camphor, geranium or ginger.*
- Cramp — *basil, cypress, geranium, ginger or marjoram.*
- Dry, flaky skin — *lavender.*
- Eczema, dry — *chamomile, lavender or geranium.*
- Eczema, weeping — *bergamot or juniper.*
- Fevers — *lavender, eucalyptus, melissa (lemon balm), peppermint or chamomile.*
- Grazes, cuts and minor wounds — *lavender, eucalyptus or thyme. For infected wounds use tea-tree, chamomile, lavender, eucalyptus or thyme.*
- Headaches — *lavender, chamomile, marjoram or peppermint.* Relieve tension headaches by putting a few drops of lavender oil in a bowl of warm water, dipping a handkerchief in it, then wringing out the handkerchief and applying it to the back of the neck.
- Insect bites — *lavender, chamomile, eucalyptus, melissa (lemon balm) or thyme.*
- Itchy skin — *chamomile.*
- Muscles, stiff and aching — *rosemary, thyme, lavender or eucalyptus.*
- Neuralgia — *chamomile or geranium.*
- Prickly heat — *chamomile, geranium or lavender.*
- Psoriasis — *bergamot or lavender.*
- Rash — *lavender or chamomile.*
- Rheumatism — *rosemary, oregano or thyme.*
- Sprains and strains — *eucalyptus, lavender, thyme or chamomile.*
- Sunburn — *lavender or chamomile.*

# Constipation

One of the best remedies for constipation is to maintain a healthy diet with plenty of fibre and water (8 glasses a day is ideal). Breakfast cereals containing oat bran and dried, soaked fruits — such as sultanas, raisins and prunes — stimulate the bowel to function naturally. Other foods which act as laxatives include tomatoes, steamed onions, globe artichokes, apples and figs. Replacing the sugar in your diet with honey also helps.

If you need a laxative, try the following remedies.

▶ Soak 6 dried prunes and 6 dried figs overnight. Wash and chop up 1 unpeeled pear and 1 apple, and add these, along with 3 cloves and a stick of cinnamon, to a pan containing 300 ml of water. Bring to the boil and boil for 3 minutes, then reduce heat and simmer (without the lid on) for 45 minutes. Remove spices, add 2 teaspoons of honey and serve either hot or cold.

▶ This serves two, is a great breakfast to start the day with, and will keep you healthy as well as regular.

▶ ½ cup of dandelion tea morning and night.

▶ 1 glass of raw beetroot juice morning and night.

▶ Slippery elm powder is a very safe and effective natural laxative, suitable for all ages, and it is also about as nutritious as porridge. The powder is available from health food stores. Mix 1 dessertspoonful of powder with just enough fruit juice to make a thick gruel and eat it at least 3 times a day.

## CHRONIC CONSTIPATION IN OLDER PEOPLE

Take 25 ml of aloe vera juice, blended with 1 cup of warm water, 4–5 times a day.

*See also Babies.*

# Cooking with Herbs

Throughout human history, the use of herbs in food has contributed a great deal towards human health. Not only those herbs cultivated in the home garden, but also the wild plants found growing in the countryside.

The regular use of herbs will add vitamins and minerals to your diet, replace salt as a flavouring agent, help prevent flatulence, promote better digestion of food — and transform a good plain meal into a gastronomic delight. Herbs can help bridge the gap between what our bodies need and what vitamins and minerals they are in fact getting.

By including herbs and natural supplements in our diet, we will not only aid our health; we will also make eating more enjoyable. It is preferable to use fresh herbs in cooking, of course, but when this is not possible, dried or frozen herbs can be used. Remember, however, that the flavour of herbs tends to become more concentrated with drying (although not with freezing), so use dried herbs sparingly, so as not to overpower the dishes you are cooking.

Some herbs are best added at the beginning of the cooking process, others only at the last minute, as prolonged cooking will destroy their delicate flavour. Most recipes will indicate the best time to add seasonings. If a recipe doesn't say, or you're experimenting with your cooking, a rough guide is to add herbs to meatloaves, stuffings, roasts, stocks, soups and casseroles at the beginning of the cooking, and to cooked vegetables and sauces 10 minutes before the end of the cooking time. Uncooked sauces and salad dressings will be far more potent if the herbs are added and left to steep for several hours before use.

It should be noted that seasonings cooked with a dish tend to become more intense after freezing. So they should either be eaten within about 2 months of their preparation, or the herbs should be omitted altogether at the cooking stage and added only when reheating.

## WILD HERBS

Wild herbs are gradually finding their way back into the human diet. Along with their cultivated cousins, they are excellent companions in any salad and, as well as being a healthy treat, will add pizzazz to most meals. They can be juiced for health-giving drinks, taken as a tea or tonic, and included in cooking. Dried and ground into a powder, they can be used as natural spices for vegetable dishes.

In many cases, quite a number of wild plants can be found growing in and around your garden: chickweed, dandelion, fat hen, purslane, shepherd's purse, sorrel, stinging nettle and wild mustard.

Chickweed's pale green floppy stems and small leaves can be simply chopped up and added to any salad, as a winter green, or to vegetable soup. You can strip off the tiny leaves by running a fork down the stem.

Young dandelion leaves can be added to summer salads or cooked as you would spinach for winter meals, and can be used as part of the vegetable content of your diet every day. They are rich in iron, silicon, magnesium, sodium and calcium — in fact they contain almost every element necessary to maintain a healthy body function.

Fat hen is higher in vitamin A and C than its popular cultivated cousin spinach, as well as matching it closely in potassium and iron. No other green comes near it in calcium value, and the 4.5 per cent protein that it contains makes the inclusion of it in your daily diet excellent for building healthy muscles and bones. It makes the perfect addition to summer salads or winter meals.

Purslane, a common weed in most gardens during the heat of summer, outranks all greens, with the exception of parsley, in organic iron content. It makes a useful addition to green salads when many other salad greens are scarce. When the leaves are dried and ground to a powder they can be used as a vegetable garnish. The high alkalinity of this herb makes it good for acid stomachs.

Add the young leaves of shepherd's purse to salads, or steam them as a winter green.

The raw leaves of sorrel can be chopped up and added to any salad or used in vegetable soup, or as a vegetable accompaniment. However, do not use this herb every day of the week, because it does contain a lot of oxalic acid (too much of this is toxic, and can inhibit the body's ability to take up iron).

The fresh green tips of stinging nettles have tremendous health value and should be picked using gloves, then steamed like any other green vegetable. They are very nutritious, giving a daily ration of iron and copper, as well as providing a well-balanced intake of calcium, lecithin, sodium, potassium and chlorine.

Wild mustard leaves can be added to summer salads or steamed or microwaved and used as a winter green.

If you are unable to identify these plants your local library can help — there are many books with full-colour pictures to help you identify wild herbs.

## WILD HERB SALAD

This salad can be eaten on its own as a light and nutritious lunch, or as a side salad with a main evening meal.

For variety and interest, use two or more different types of lettuce torn into smallish pieces. To this add lots of watercress, alfalfa and red clover sprouts, chives, parsley, and very young dandelion leaves torn into about 2.5 cm bits. (Older, larger dandelion leaves have a bitter taste.) Then add smaller amounts of basil, dill, lemon balm and nasturtium leaves, with a very small garnish of mint, oregano and lemon thyme.

Just before serving, toss the salad in wine vinegar, or one of the many herb vinegars available from supermarkets and health food shops.

## WILD HERB GARNISH

Wild herbs can also be used as a garnish wherever you would usually use salt. Combine 1 tablespoon each of dried celery seed, thyme and oregano, toasted sesame seeds, and any one of the wild herbs previously mentioned. Ensure that they are well mixed, then reduce the mixture to a powder in a blender, with a pestle and mortar, or by rubbing it through a fine wire sieve. Store in an airtight jar (label and date the jar), and use within 12 months.

# Corns

Rub the corn with a crushed garlic clove every night, or put a sliver of garlic on the corn and hold it on your foot with sticking plaster. Another remedy is to apply freshly crushed marigold (*Calendula officinalis*) leaves to the corn morning and night until the corn disappears — hold them on with a bandage.

# Coughs

Warm, chesty coughs are a good indication that you should avoid mucus-producing foods, such as dairy products, fried foods, meat and white bread. Replace dairy foods with soya bean substitutes, and include barley, rice, cabbage, carrots, zucchinis, broccoli, lettuce, spinach, garlic, pears and citrus fruits in your diet.

Dry coughs need a moist diet, with lots of salads and lightly cooked green vegetables. A ticklish or persistent cough can be soothed by sucking on a horehound cough lozenge, as needed.

To make the cough lozenges, boil equal parts of the fresh herb juice and sugar until it sets, then cut it into squares. Store in an airtight jar and keep moisture free.

The following remedies also help relieve a cough:

▶ Mix the juice from ½ lemon with 2 tablespoons of honey and administer every 15 minutes.
▶ Take 1 teaspoon of onion syrup every now and then (*see Onion, Onion Syrup*).
▶ Grind 6 almonds into a fine meal, add 1 cup of warm water, the juice of 1 lemon and honey to taste. Store in the refrigerator and drink 1 tablespoonful every now and then.
▶ To ease a dry cough, mix 2 drops each of eucalyptus oil and lemon oil with 2 tablespoons of honey. Dilute 1 teaspoon of the mixture in a wineglass of warm water and sip slowly.

## NATURAL DECONGESTANT

If you are plagued by a nagging cough, try the following natural decongestant. Chop up 6 garlic cloves and slice 1 onion into rings. Spread the ingredients out on a small shallow ovenproof or microwave tray (do not use metal or aluminium, since both these materials can react unfavourably with the ingredients), and cover thickly with honey. Seal the tray tightly with plastic wrap, place it carefully inside a plastic bag, seal the open end, and leave it in the refrigerator overnight.

Strain the mixture into a sterilised glass jar, pushing down on the garlic and onion with the back of a spoon until the honey stops dripping. You will find that the honey has lost considerable viscosity and runs very freely. Take 1 teaspoon of the mixture every 2–3 hours or whenever needed.

*See also Thyme.*

# Cuts and Grazes

Bathe the area with an antiseptic made by dissolving 5 drops of lavender oil and 2 drops of tea-tree oil in 500 ml of warm water, then cover with a suitable dressing. Place 3 drops of lavender oil or calendula ointment (available from chemists, health food stores and supermarkets) on a piece of gauze and place it over the affected area, renewing twice a day.

Add 2–3 drops of tea-tree or lavender oil to a bowl of warm water for an excellent antiseptic. Wash the wound thoroughly then apply the tea-tree or lavender solution with a clean cotton wool ball 3 times a day.

Undiluted apple cider vinegar is also an excellent antiseptic.

*See also Tea-Tree Oil, Thyme.*

# Cystitis

Drink a glass of raw beetroot juice morning and night if you are troubled by a urinary tract infection. Bicarbonate of soda is also a helpful first aid remedy for a sudden attack of cystitis. Add 1 level teaspoon of bicarbonate of soda to a glass of water, and drink once an hour for 3 hours to relieve acute symptoms.

Another helpful remedy is old-fashioned barley water. Barley is well known for its anti-inflammatory action on the genito-urinary tract. To make your own barley water, simmer 50 g of unrefined barley (from health food stores) in 1 litre of water for 40 minutes. Cool, strain and drink over 24 hours.

If the problem persists, consult your health practitioner.

# D

## Dandelion

Dandelion (*Taraxacum officinale*) is a virtual storehouse of active substances — vitamins, minerals, enzymes, proteins, and other valuable elements — making it a wholesome plant food. The leaf can be taken as a tea, or the root can be dried, roasted and ground and drunk as a coffee substitute. Dandelion has a general fortifying effect on the body, and is said to improve digestion, have a beneficial effect on the liver, kidneys and gall bladder, and be excellent for treating constipation and piles. Freshly squeezed juice from the hollow stem, applied externally, can be a cure for warts.

Taken regularly as a tea, dandelion adds a healthy bloom to the complexion; it can also be used daily as a general tonic. You can buy dandelion leaf tea or dandelion root coffee substitute from health food stores.

*See also Coffee Substitute.*

## Dandruff

Those telltale flakes of dead skin cells scattered on your shoulders are a good indication that your head and hair are in bad condition. Even if you brush your hair thoroughly in the morning and brush your shoulders before leaving the house, by the middle of the day those embarrassing white flakes will be back again, making a mess of your appearance and, quite often, your social life.

Often food allergies and sugary diets can promote dandruff. Cut down on excessively spicy foods, too much fat and sugar, very starchy white flour products and alcohol (as far as possible), particularly spirits. Eat plenty of raw vegetables and fruits, vegetable oils and nuts, lean meat and fish. Correct eating goes a long way towards improving this condition.

Rosemary or nutmeg oils massaged into the scalp can also be effective in controlling dandruff. Essential oils will usually help you get to the root of the problem and banish it once and for all, and can be used in conjunction with the following after-shampoo conditioning oil: put 1 teaspoon of dried rosemary or 6 sprigs of fresh rosemary into a ceramic bowl, add boiling water, cover, steep for 12 hours, then strain and blend 180 ml of this infusion with 30 ml each of almond and castor oil and 10 drops of rosemary essential oil. Store in an old shampoo bottle.

To use, wet hair thoroughly and massage conditioning oil well into scalp and hair with fingertips for about 2 minutes. Rinse out with clean, warm water.

A small amount of warmed olive oil can also be used to treat dry-scalp dandruff. Simply massage well into the scalp and leave for about 15 minutes, then wash out.

An after-shampoo astringent rinse that is suitable for all hair types, and that will close the pores and remove dandruff, can be made from rosemary and cider vinegar. Put 1 cup of fresh rosemary leaves in an enamel or stainless steel saucepan, add 1 litre of water, bring to the boil, simmer for 15 minutes, remove from heat and allow to steep until cool. Strain through muslin and blend with 125 ml of cider vinegar. Store in an airtight bottle. After shampooing and rinsing, massage a small amount of the liquid well into your scalp.

Dandruff will also respond very well to this scalp conditioning treatment: blend together 5 drops each of jojoba oil, evening primrose oil and carrot oil and 3 drops of rosemary essential oil with 30 ml of slightly warmed castor oil. Store in an airtight, amber-coloured glass bottle for no longer than 2 months. Dip your fingertips into the mixture and massage into your scalp every night before you go to bed.

To warm the oil before use, stand it in a container of hot water for a few minutes.

Most cases of dandruff will respond well to home treatments; combining the external applications with a good internal regime should give positive results quite quickly. If you find that modification to your diet and the use of homemade herbal preparations do not work, and you are suffering scalp inflammation and bleeding or other severe irritation, you should see a doctor, medical herbalist, dermatologist or trichologist.

*See also Hair, Jojoba.*

# Depression

*See Eating for Health and Energy (Grapes, Potatoes), Stress and Tension.*

# Detoxification

Overindulgence in food and alcohol, bad eating habits and smoking can all pollute the body with toxins. Include the following herbs and vegetables in your diet to help rid your body of harmful toxins: celery, parsley, sage, salad burnet, rosemary, fennel, thyme, sunflower seeds, radishes, beetroot, watermelon and sesame seeds. To help cleanse your system, dilute 10 ml of apple cider vinegar in a glass of warm water, add 2 small pinches of cayenne pepper, mix well and drink twice a day.

*See Fasting, Herbal Detox, Overindulgence.*

# Diabetes

Diet is important with this condition. Eat plenty of cabbage, celery, green vegetables, mandarins, parsley, olives, soya beans and sunflower seeds.

A cup of nettle tea daily is also helpful.

**Warning:** *Molasses must not be taken by anyone suffering from diabetes.*

# Diarrhoea

Take ½ teaspoon of nutmeg several times during the day. Drink 1 glass of freshly prepared vegetable juice consisting of equal quantities of carrot, celery and apple juice each morning. For best digestion, sip slowly.

Avoid leafy green vegetables, but eat plenty of pumpkin, carrots and zucchinis, plus apples, mandarins, pears and tangerines. Mandarins are excellent for calming irritated intestines.

Slippery elm powder is also an excellent, safe and nutritious remedy. Mix 1 dessertspoon of the powder thoroughly with enough fruit juice to make a sloppy paste and take 3 times a day.

Other causes of chronic diarrhoea are high doses of vitamin C — cut down your daily dosage — and a high intake of dried fruits, figs and rhubarb. After diarrhoea has ceased, eat some grated raw apple to restore your bowel function to normal.

If you continually suffer from chronic diarrhoea, you should check with your health practitioner as to the cause. It can quite easily be caused by food allergies, lactose intolerance, colitis, coeliac disease or diverticulitis.

## CHILDREN

Fresh apple juice, bananas or brown rice water, and diluted soups should be given to avoid dehydration. Brown rice water can be sweetened with honey to make it more palatable. Avoid dairy products and soft drinks, as they will only aggravate the problem. If the diarrhoea is severe or prolonged, seek medical help. Diarrhoea in children should not be treated as a minor ailment; children under 3 must be referred to your family doctor straightaway. This condition can become critical in children very quickly. Should diarrhoea be a continuing problem, have the child checked out for food allergies or food intolerances.

---

*See also Eating for Health and Energy (Carrots), Medicinal Food (Apples, Carrots, Pears).*

# Diet

A healthy diet should consist of lots of raw vegetables, fresh fruit, nuts and sprouted seeds. If vegetables are to be cooked, steam them until just tender or bake them. Avoid animal protein, white sugar and white flour, all of which are very mucus-forming.

Vegetable soups are nutritious and healthy, because the nutrients that are cooked out of the vegetables are retained in the liquid.

A complete change to only fresh fruits, raw vegetables and living food would no doubt be difficult at first, as a lifetime of bad eating habits is hard to change. But it is possible. When gradually changing your diet, there are a number of basic nutritional guidelines to follow. These will allow the cleansing process to take place more effectively.

First and foremost, avoid refined and processed foods.

| | |
|---|---|
| Dairy | Pasteurised products are completely useless, as this process destroys enzymes, amino acids and vitamins, causing an excessive build-up of mucus in the body. |
| Eggs | Eat only fresh farm eggs laid by free-range chickens. They are more nutritious and far more easily assimilated. *See also Eggs*. |
| Fruit | Use freely, whole and unpeeled whenever possible. It is the most perfect food for humankind, and the easiest to digest. |
| Nuts and grains | Excellent food, but they assimilate better if sprouted first. |
| Oils and fats | Unsalted butter and olive oil — no others. |
| Protein | Always use meat sparingly, especially red meat. Fresh fish or chicken is a far better choice, provided that it is organically grown and only included in meals once or twice a week. Never eat red meat after 1 pm. It is important to allow the digestive system to do its job and then rest when the body is resting. |

| | |
|---|---|
| Salt | Only use sea salt or salt substitute. |
| Sweeteners | Use absolutely no sugar in your diet. Substitute raw honey or molasses. |
| Vegetables | Eat raw vegetables whenever possible. If they are to be cooked, steam them until tender, or bake. Potatoes or other roots can be cooked in about 6 mm of water in the bottom of a glass baking dish at 180°C for about 1½ hours. |
| Water | Drink plenty of fresh water which is free of chemical treatments such as chlorine and fluoride. Low-salt natural mineral water makes an ideal substitute for pure water. However, you can make your own biochemically free water easily and quickly. *See Water.* |

When cooking, use only glass, porcelain, enamel or stainless steel utensils. Cook at low temperatures, and only for as long as it takes to break down fibre or starch. It's best to steam green vegetables and cook potatoes and root vegetables, including squash, pumpkin, etc., as described above. Allow food to cool to body temperature before you eat it, and add sprouts, or other living food, just before serving.

# Dietary Substitutes

As creatures of habit we become used to certain foods in our daily diet, and quite often when (for health reasons) a major change to this routine has to be made, we are left feeling devastated. A change in our diet does not have to be devastating, as there are tasty and healthy alternatives to many of our staples. In fact you may even find the natural alternatives preferable to the food they're replacing.

## BEVERAGES

*Coffee — see Coffee Substitute.*

*Tea — see Herbal Teas.*

# DAIRY SUBSTITUTES

### Dairy-free Butter

Use the following herbal spread:

*dried herbs of your choice or garlic*
*4 tablespoons food yeast*
*1 teaspoon powdered kelp*
*olive oil*

Mince the garlic or reduce the dried herbs to a powder by rubbing
them through a fine wire sieve.
Combine all ingredients, using sufficient olive oil to create a butter-like
consistency, and process in a blender. Store in a suitable airtight
container in the refrigerator.

### Dairy-free Cheese

This makes a soft cottage cheese-like cheese substitute.

*1 cup (125 g) unsalted cashew nuts*
*⅔ cup (120 g) sunflower seeds*
*1 cup (250 ml) water*
*dried herbs to taste*

Process nuts and seeds in a blender until fine, doing small amounts at
a time. Fold water in slowly to make a smooth, thick batter.
Ferment by allowing the mixture to stand for 12–24 hours at 20–25°C,
until it has a fluffy consistency. Add the herbs and refrigerate for
several hours before using.

### Dairy-free Cream

*½ cup (90 g) almonds*
*1 cup (250 ml) water*
*1 tablespoon honey*
*¼ cup (60 ml) cold-pressed corn oil*

Chop the almonds into small pieces and process with water and
honey in a blender, then add the oil in a thin stream.

### *Milk Substitute*

Soya milk, either fresh or powdered, is a healthy substitute for dairy milk. Fruit juices are delicious on breakfast cereals and muesli, and can be used in baking in place of milk.

You can make your own seed/nut milk from sunflower or sesame seeds or almond or cashew nuts.

*½ cup (90 g) selected seeds*
*1–2 cups (250–500 ml) water*

Place the seeds in a blender and grind them, then add water and process at high speed till smooth and creamy.

Use as is to pour over cereals, blend with fruit and/or fruit juice to make smoothies, or strain to make a thinner milk for use in beverages, such as coffee substitutes.

### *Sunflower Milk Smoothie*

*4 cups (800 g) sunflower seeds*
*3 or 4 bananas, peeled and sliced*
*a few slices of fresh pawpaw*
*flesh of 1 or 2 passionfruit*

Combine all ingredients in a blender and process until smooth.

## SALT SUBSTITUTE

*See Salt (Herbal Salt Substitute).*

## SUGAR SUBSTITUTES

Ideal replacements for sugar are:

- ▶ Molasses — contains more minerals than the same quantity of honey
- ▶ Honey
- ▶ Treacle — a more refined form of molasses
- ▶ Dates — very sweet, and can be used in breakfast foods, such as porridge

▶ Dried fruits such as apricots and sultanas — can be added to either raw or cooked food

*See also Eating for Health and Energy, Garlic.*

# Digestion

Many of the herbs best known and most often used for flavouring and seasoning also stimulate the flow of digestive juices in the stomach and intestines. Classic herb and food partnerships in cooking reflect this: rosemary helps the digestion of fatty lamb; fennel assists the digestion of oily fish; horseradish aids the digestion of beef.

Aromatic seeds such as aniseed, cardamom, caraway, dill and fennel are also useful digestives. A tablespoon of ground aniseed boiled in a cup of milk and drunk twice a day will improve digestion. To increase the flow of saliva, add 1 teaspoon of cardamom to the aniseed drink and take it ½ hour before meals.

*See also Dill Water, Indigestion, Onion.*

# Dill Water

Dill water helps the body absorb food and aids digestion. It is also excellent for calming hiccups, and will help induce restful sleep. It is free of harmful effects and can be given safely to young children.

*25 g dill seed*
*300 ml hot water*
*1 tablespoon honey*

Crush the dill seed with a mortar and pestle, or with the back of a metal spoon on a chopping board, then soak for 3–4 hours in the water. Strain and sweeten with the honey. Sip a small amount after meals twice a day.

# Dizziness

See Lavender (Lavender Tea), Menopause (Cucumber Juice), Sunstroke.

# Dong Quai

Often called the 'female ginseng', dong quai (*Angelica sinensis*) is a member of the carrot family. The root is rich in phytoestrogens and plant oestrogenic substances that have a normalising effect on a woman's hormonal fluctuations. Dong quai will help regulate the female menstrual cycle and ease the effects of menopause. It can also be used as a reproductive tonic during all fertile cycles of a woman's life.

Tablets and capsules are available from health food stores, but you will have to consult a herbalist if you want a stronger dose, in the form of a tincture or liquid extract.

# Dry Bathing

Dry bathing consists of brushing all parts of the body below the neck — with the exception of the delicate breast areas in women — with a loofah. Go very gently and lightly on the paler, softer areas of the stomach and the inside areas of the arms and legs. Over the rest of the body, use a gentle yet firm pressure, and brush in a rhythmic circular motion.

Each morning when you get up, brush for 5–10 minutes to stimulate your circulation and rid your body of accumulated dead cells and toxins. Finish off by gently applying almond or apricot kernel oil all over your body. Leave for 10 minutes, then towel off the excess with a vigorous rub.

*See also Bathing.*

# E

## Earache

Gently heat 2 chopped cloves of garlic in 2 teaspoons of olive oil. Strain the oil through clean muslin or cheesecloth and allow it to cool until it is just warm. Insert a few drops of the warm oil in the offending ear, and plug the outer ear with cotton wool. If pain persists, consult your health practitioner.

## Eating for Health and Energy

The idea that you can eat whatever you like as long as you pop a few vitamin pills is a fallacy. It just doesn't work. Your way of eating largely determines whether you are brimming with energy or dragging yourself through the day and evening.

Everything we eat gives us energy. It's just that some foods are better than others for boosting our energy supplies. Carbohydrates are the best source of energy, so don't feel guilty about an extra serving of potatoes or rice.

From a nutritional point of view, the best type of carbohydrates are the natural sugars that are found in fruit and vegetables, and complex carbohydrates such as bread, pasta, rice, potatoes, cereals and grains. Raw fruits and vegetables are the key to eating for energy, though. For maximum vitality, 50–75 per cent of what you eat should be raw.

A diet high in raw foods has been credited with stimulating healing, rejuvenation, an improved mental and emotional state and enhanced athletic performance. Fruit, especially, is the most perfect food for humankind. In taste it is delicious, and it is the easiest food to digest, the least mucus-inducing, and will open your sinuses to improve breathing.

Because fruit is high in citric and other acids, it has an acid pH reaction in the digestion. Yet because it also has a high proportion of alkali-forming minerals, fruit has an alkaline reaction in the bloodstream. This helps neutralise the waste products of metabolism, which are always acid. Fruit acts as a natural laxative, promoting the secretory action of the liver, pancreas and other secretory glands.

Whenever possible, eat only organically grown fruit, which has been picked when it is almost ready to drop from the tree. It is then at peak ripeness and contains the most juice. For ease of digestion it is far better to juice the fruit than to eat it whole. Fruit that has not been organically grown, and which has been picked unripe or treated with chemicals, should be avoided.

The antioxidants found in fruit and vegetables can also help prevent a wide variety of degenerative illnesses and protect the body against the harmful effects of pollution and ultraviolet light, which can damage body cells. These include beta carotene (which makes vitamin A in the body), and vitamins C and E — these are sometimes known as the ACE vitamins. But antioxidants aren't the only thing in fruit and vegetables that are good for us. Scientists have now discovered phytochemicals: obscure but naturally occurring chemicals with an equally powerful disease-fighting ability.

Every plant contains hundreds of phytochemicals that fight the damaging effects of sunlight and oxygen. It now seems that they can be beneficial to humans, too; they are believed to be instrumental in the fight against cancer.

There are yet other reasons to eat plenty of fruit and vegetables: fibre, for example. Dietary fibre is a carbohydrate made up of the material which forms the cell walls of plants. There are two types of fibre: insoluble fibre, such as wheat bran, and soluble fibre, such as fruits and legumes. Insoluble fibre cannot be digested by body enzymes, so it passes through the body as roughage. It is essential for a properly functioning bowel. It holds water and shortens the time taken for food waste to leave the body. Lack of sufficient insoluble fibre in your diet will cause constipation.

Soluble fibre is easily digested and is processed by bacteria to produce valuable acids. It is necessary to help control blood sugar and cholesterol levels. Research has shown that lack of fibre in the human diet may lead to conditions such as piles, obesity, diverticulitis and even bowel cancer. It is important, therefore, to maintain a well-balanced diet that provides adequate fibre, and not to get enough fibre by simply sprinkling large amounts of raw bran over breakfast cereal.

The best way to start the day, and to ensure that you receive an adequate supply of both types of fibre, is with a good breakfast of whole cereals, then a snack of washed, unpeeled fruit mid-morning and mid-afternoon, and salads and raw, or slightly cooked, vegetables with your lunch and evening meal. Eat wholemeal bread, rice and pastas instead of the refined varieties, and include plenty of legumes, nuts and dried fruit in your diet. Do this and you will feel healthy, vibrant, vital and bursting with energy.

There are also, however, certain foods that, because they are a perfectly packed balance of nutritional value, are especially easy for the body to assimilate. Incorporating these foods in your diet will also boost your energy levels and give you an overall feeling of wellbeing. These foods are:

## ALMONDS

An important source of the minerals zinc, magnesium, potassium and iron. A handful of nuts can quickly transform any light salad into a well-balanced meal.

It is important, when eating almonds with any meal, to also include foods rich in vitamin C, because almonds contain oxalic and phytic acid, which can prevent the absorption of this vitamin.

## APRICOTS

The brighter the fruit the greater the amount of beta-carotene it contains. Dried apricots are high in vitamin A and make an energy-packed addition to any breakfast cereal.

## AVOCADOS

This fruit is almost a complete food, rich in potassium and vitamin A.

## BARLEY

Apart from its very high mineral content, barley has lots of calcium, potassium and B complex vitamins, making it especially useful in combating stress and fatigue.

## BEETROOT

This is an excellent vegetable for aiding digestion, especially if eaten raw and grated, served with grated apple and carrot, and dressed with lemon juice and olive oil.

## BROCCOLI

Broccoli is rich in vitamin C, iron, beta-carotene and folic acid. Like all green vegetables, it is best cooked by steaming, so as to preserve most of its nutrients.

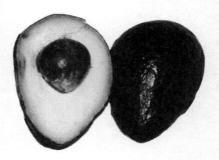

## CARROTS

A single carrot will supply all your vitamin A needs for a day. Nibbling on a carrot stick is a much healthier snack than salted nuts, pretzels or crisps.

Carrot juice is rich in beta-carotene and numerous other beneficial substances, which affect (in particular) the liver and the gall bladder. This juice helps regulate the digestive process and rectify constipation and diarrhoea.

However, carrot juice must be taken in moderation, as an excess of beta-carotene will kill vitamin D in your body. One glassful each morning on rising is the recommended dose. In fact, limit yourself to only one glassful in total of vegetable juice per day, to let your digestive juices act upon the complex materials.

## CELERY

Rich in vitamins A, B and C, celery helps combat diseases of the liver, kidneys and urinary tract. It also helps eliminate waste via the urine, due to the effect it has on the kidneys.

## CIDER VINEGAR

This is unusually high in potassium, calcium, phosphorus, sodium and trace elements, and has the ability to increase oxygenation of the blood, improve the metabolism, strengthen the digestion and increase clotting of the blood.

## GARLIC

Garlic is especially useful for cleansing toxins from your bloodstream, nourishing your nerves and increasing glandular secretions, helping digestion and cleansing stale mucus from your tissues.

---

*See also Garlic.*

## GRAPES

Grapes are very cleansing and regenerating. Fasting by eating only grapes and drinking water for 2 days is a well-known method of detoxifying the body. Grapes are an ideal food when you are convalescing, or suffering from fatigue or depression.

## KELP

This is an excellent source of iodine. It protects your body from radioactivity in the atmosphere, such as strontium 90, that contributes to early ageing.

Kelp is rich in vitamin B complex, vitamins D, E and K, and magnesium and calcium. It is particularly good for the health of your hair and nails.

## LECITHIN

Lecithin helps you maintain a healthy nervous system and is vital in resisting stress.

Consuming lecithin daily means that body fats are converted into energy far more quickly, and existing fat deposits will slowly disperse. It will also help break up cholesterol so that it can pass through the artery walls, and it is reputed to increase immunity to virus infection.

## PUMPKIN, SUNFLOWER AND SESAME SEEDS

These three seeds make a protein and vitamin-packed addition to salads and fruits, and are excellent for your hair and skin, as well as your general health.

Pumpkin seeds are rich in B vitamins, phosphorus, iron and zinc. Sesame seeds are rich in magnesium and potassium and have been used for many years to treat fatigue, insomnia and sexual dysfunction. They also contain more calcium than milk, cheese or nuts, and are a good source of vitamin E. Sunflower seeds are rich in iron, the B complex vitamins, magnesium and zinc.

Add equal proportions of each seed to a blender or coffee grinder, reduce them to a powder, then sprinkle it over your food.

# MOLASSES

A tablespoon of blackstrap molasses supplies as much calcium as a glass of milk, as much iron as 9 eggs, more potassium than any other food, and a balanced supply of B complex vitamins. It is also rich in vitamin E, magnesium and copper, and is an excellent iron source for women who tend to be anaemic.

Because molasses is an alkali-forming food, it helps maintain a proper alkaline/acid balance in the body, and contributes to the overall health of your skin and hair.

A tablespoon of molasses and the juice of $\frac{1}{2}$ lemon dissolved in a mug of hot water is a good way to start the day.

---

**Warning:** *Molasses must not be taken by anyone suffering from diabetes.*

# OATS

Oats are a good source of iron and a uniquely soothing food for the nerves. You can get your daily ration from your porridge, if that's what you prefer, and it will give you a good start to the day. Add fresh seasonal fruit and some wheat germ and you have a super get-up-and-go breakfast.

Oats are also very high in calcium, potassium and magnesium, as well as lots of B complex vitamins, which are essential for the health of your nervous system. Eaten on a regular basis, they also help lower cholesterol levels.

# POTATOES

A potato is not only an ideal carbohydrate; it also contains vitamins A, C, B1, B6, niacin, iron, potassium and fibre. Potatoes are known to have a soporific effect, because they contain a substance very much like chloroform. Research has suggested that this may cause contentment and lift depression, because the brain chemistry is altered in a similar way to therapy with drugs.

## SPROUTED GRAINS

Sprouted grains are living food that will grow in any climate, and that rival meat in nutritional value. Unlike most vegetables, they are eaten at the peak of their freshness — when they are still growing. They are rich in vitamins A, C, D, E, K and B complex, in calcium, phosphorus, potassium, magnesium, iron, high-quality protein and an amazing number of enzymes.

Sprouts are highly nutritious, extremely low in kilojoules, and produce more efficient digestion and metabolism of food into energy.

*See Living Foods for information on how to grow your own sprouts.*

## SPIRULINA

Spirulina is an excellent source of protein and contains vitamin B12, folic acid and chlorophyll, making it useful in the treatment of anaemia. It also contains the amino acid phenylalanine, which is helpful in weight control. This amino acid is transformed into a brain neurotransmitter substance that controls appetite, energy levels and moods.

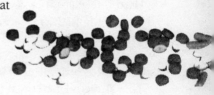

Spirulina is available in tablet form from health food stores. Follow the directions on the bottle.

## WHEAT GERM

Not only is wheat germ the richest source of vitamin E, it is also rich in magnesium, copper, manganese, calcium and phosphorus. A tablespoonful of wheat germ sprinkled over your breakfast cereal will provide almost your entire daily requirement of iron. It is also a superb source of protein, but it is rich in fat, so eat no more than 1 tablespoon a day.

*See also Garlic, Iron, Living Foods, Medicinal Food.*

# Echinacea

Should you ever get the chance to play word association with a herbalist, try 'colds and flu'. Most likely, their response will be 'echinacea'. It is one of the most popular plants used by herbalists, and over recent years it has received a considerable amount of attention, especially for its reputed ability to boost the immune system.

Commonly known as 'cone flower', echinacea (*Echinacea angustifolia*) is one of the most medicinal of all the herbs, and has long been used as a blood purifier and to help build up resistance to infection. Native Mexicans used to bind its leaves around wounds to promote healing, to prevent infection and to stop pain; Native Americans used it as a snakebite remedy.

It has a long history of use as an immuno-stimulant and natural antitoxin, but how — or how much of — this herb stimulates the immune system is still undetermined. However, modern scientific research appears to support its immuno-stimulant properties, along with its value as an external antiseptic.

Used internally, it is said to help prevent and ease influenza and to reduce the frequency and severity of attacks of herpes simplex; when used as an external antiseptic it will help slow-healing wounds. The juice from the fresh flowers can also be used externally to treat bacterial infections.

This attractive perennial herb can be grown in home gardens in most parts of Australia. The beautiful purple petals that radiate from its dark cone-shaped centre look a little like Black-eyed Susan. Its seeds can be used in a herbal tea to treat all sorts of infections, fevers and bites.

Echinacea is available from health food stores in tablet or capsule form, or as a herbal tea, and can be taken internally as a botanical antibiotic. Its reputation for stimulating the immune system makes it an excellent tonic for treating coughs, colds, flu and other infections, as well as for easing allergies.

Many herbalists now recommend taking a daily preventive dose of this herb to enhance the immune system and lessen the chance of catching colds and flu. However, follow the directions for taking the tablets, capsules or tea, or the directions of your health practitioner.

During winter you may find that echinacea is the perfect natural choice to help build up your immune system so you don't catch a cold, or to alleviate its symptoms. To make your own echinacea herbal tea, steep 1 teaspoon of the dried seeds in 1 cup of boiling water for 10 minutes. Strain, reheat, sweeten with honey if desired, and drink as hot as possible 3–4 times a day when suffering from a cold or flu; or drink 1 cup of the tea morning and night as a preventive.

*See also Antiseptic, Colds, Fever.*

# Eczema

Eczema is the name given to a number of similar skin complaints, all of which are usually characterised by tightness and excess dryness of the skin. In severe cases it can lead to cracking, and bleeding or weeping of the skin, accompanied by continual itchiness.

In many cases the cause is a particular substance, such as strong or highly perfumed soap, washing powder and liquid, cheaper costume jewellery, cats, dogs, powder paints, cement. Diet and stress can also play an important role in this condition. Avoid cow's milk — goat's milk is an excellent substitute — and refined, processed foods. Take plenty of wholemeal flour products, sprouts (especially mung beans and alfalfa), fresh fruit and vegetables, dried beans, lentils, soya beans, nuts, yeast, B vitamins, honey, and sunflower and sesame seeds.

Try to find a way of relaxing to relieve tension. Set aside a little time each day to do absolutely nothing. Just relax: stare into space, watch the waves at the beach, or watch the wind in the trees. In fact do anything that allows you to turn off. Join a yoga or meditation class, or simply go for a daily walk or bike ride (*see Stress and Tension*).

Cleansers and herbal applications also play an important part in treating eczema-affected skin:

73

## CLEANSING THE SKIN

You will need 2 small muslin bath bags. Fill the first bag with any combination of the following herbs — chamomile, comfrey, calendula, marshmallow or lime flowers — and hang it from the tap so that the water gushes through it as the bath fills. Fill the second bag with finely ground oatmeal, tie the top tightly, immerse the bag in water, and rub it gently over your face, body and limbs.

Adding 2 teaspoons of almond or sunflower oil to your bathwater will not only moisturise and soothe your skin, it will often also help stop your skin tightening up too much.

You may also find that reducing the number of baths or showers you take will help alleviate some of the itchiness and skin cracking.

## SOAPWORT CLEANSER

A decoction of fresh or dried soapwort (roots, leaves and flowers) makes an excellent cleanser for this type of skin condition, and is one of the gentlest forms of soap for any skin type.

Add 30 g of the chopped herb to an enamel or stainless steel pan, cover with 1 litre of water, bring to the boil, cover, and simmer for 30 minutes. Cool, strain and store in a sterilised bottle in the refrigerator. Use within 7 days (dispose of sooner if it starts to smell off).

Use it in the shower or bath. This lotion is excellent for scalp eczema and can also be used as a shampoo.

## TOPICAL TREATMENTS:

▶ Apply aloe vera leaf jelly, fresh strawberry pulp or fresh pulped grapes to the affected area.
▶ A mixture of yogurt and carrot, when applied to eczema, will usually relieve the itching very quickly. Finely grate a small carrot and mix it thoroughly with a small tub (100 g) of plain yogurt. Store in the refrigerator for a week before using, and keep refrigerated when not in use. Dab gently onto affected areas.

▶ As a first aid measure, apply a few drops of jojoba oil to the affected area.

*See also Itchiness, Jojoba, Psoriasis, Rashes, Skin Irritations.*

# Eggs

Although eggs are a good source of protein and rich in vitamins A and B complex, as well as many essential minerals, they do have a high cholesterol content. In fact, they contain more cholesterol than most foods in the human diet.

It is important to note that eggs produced commercially are lower in vitamins and minerals than those obtained from free-range hens. A further downside to commercial egg production is the amount of chemicals absorbed into the eggs from the intestines of the egg-laying chickens, which are living in unnatural conditions and being fed synthetic foods. If eggs are to be included in your diet, they should be the freshest and most natural possible. If it is not possible to keep a few chooks in your backyard, seek out a source of eggs from hens living in natural conditions.

The most nutritious way to serve eggs is to separate the yolk and white, discard the white, and then serve the yolk over hot, steamed vegetables. This gives an added flavour to the vegetables, and the egg yolk does not suffer any vitamin or protein loss from high temperatures. It is also wise to limit your weekly intake of eggs to help keep your cholesterol level in check. Four to five eggs per week should be the maximum; this should be further reduced to no more than 3 a week if meat is included in your diet.

Eggs are not essential to the human diet. Nuts and lightly sprouted seeds and pulses are a more nutritious source of natural protein.

# Energy Breakfast

As well as providing nutrition and much needed energy throughout the day, this energy breakfast has definite healing properties. It is excellent when recovering from illness and as a dietary support for any illness, especially anxiety-related conditions.

### Individual Serving

*2 handfuls sprouted wheat*
*1 handful each of sultanas and raisins, plus soakwater*
*1 piece apple, finely chopped*
*1 piece seasonal fruit, finely diced*
*1 tablespoon fresh cream*
*1 handful mixed nuts, ground*
*powdered cinnamon*
*powdered vanilla bean*

Soak and sprout wheat seed. To avoid the sprout taste, eat the seed once the germ is 2–3 mm in length, no longer.
Soak the sultanas and raisins overnight and reserve the soakwater.
Mix the wheat sprouts, dried fruit plus soakwater, fruit, cream and nuts together and sprinkle with a pinch of powdered cinnamon and of vanilla bean.

---

*See also Eating for Health and Energy.*

# Energy Fruit Salad

Fresh fruit is one of the best foods for humans. It is the easiest to digest, and is the highest in natural moisture and energy-producing nutrients. This high-energy fruit salad is a complete lunch meal in itself, supplying abundant protein, vitamins and minerals.

Combine in a bowl, mixing lightly, the following ingredients: 1 large banana, peeled and diced, 1 large apple, diced, 1 large pear, diced, 6 apricots (fresh or sun-dried), diced, 1 small mango, peeled, seeded and diced (or seasonal equivalent), 50 g sun-dried dates, seeded and halved, 5 g seedless raisins. Serve immediately.

To turn your fruit salad into an extra-healthy dessert alternative add the following Tofu Cream Whip as topping. Place 2 tablespoons of cold-pressed vegetable oil (not olive oil), 1 block of tofu, 1 teaspoon of honey and any fresh or dried soaked fruit in a blender and process until the mixture has a creamy texture. Fold in a little apple juice, maintaining the creaminess of the tofu whip, and pour over your energy fruit salad or fresh seasonal fruit of your choice.

*See also Eating for Health and Energy, High-Protein Mixed Salad.*

# Exercise

Why is exercise so important? Simply, exercise burns up kilojoules and raises your body's metabolic rate for 24–48 hours afterwards. However, before embarking on an exercise regime make sure you choose a programme or sport that fits your lifestyle. Once you have chosen your exercise regime, do it regularly.

For successful weight loss through exercise, you need to expend energy in a way that is 'aerobic' — in other words, you need to engage in an activity that increases the oxygen needs of your body, thereby exercising your heart and lungs. An exercise programme that uses the large muscles of the body — thighs, trunk and shoulders — over an extended period is an excellent form of aerobic body conditioning.

When you exercise 'aerobically' on a regular basis and maintain a well-balanced, healthy diet, you may also notice that the scales show no weight loss at all; in some circumstances you may even show a weight gain. There is no need to hit the panic button, nor become discouraged. As you exercise and lose fat you will be replacing it with muscle, which is heavier, plus your muscle-to-fat ratio will have increased. Instead of relying on your scales, rely on a measuring tape and on how your clothes fit.

When choosing an exercise programme, find an activity that is convenient, enjoyable and can be sustained for at least 30 minutes or more as a continuous movement. Start at a beginner's level, and as you develop stamina and condition gradually increase your activity. Most importantly, tailor your exercise programme to your physical condition and lifestyle. If you are unsure about what's best for you, or you are unfit, check with your health practitioner before you embark on any vigorous exercise regime.

## THE BENEFITS OF EXERCISE

▶ It increases the metabolic rate, which accounts for some 70 per cent of kilojoule expenditure.
▶ Muscle strength and joint flexibility are improved. This is important in terms of fighting osteoarthritis.
▶ The risk of bone fracture, and the development of osteoporosis in women, is reduced.
▶ It helps reduce blood pressure.
▶ It helps lower blood cholesterol, including a portion of the dangerous LDL-cholesterol fraction.
▶ It reduces blood glucose levels; diabetics will benefit, as exercise increases the effectiveness of insulin.

For a better activity regime:

▶ Walk more often, instead of catching a bus or driving a car.
▶ Instead of taking a lift, walk up the stairs.
▶ Invest in an exercise bike. Pedal daily while you read or watch television.
▶ Go for a daily walk — in the evening, no later than 2 hours before bed, is a good time.
▶ Take regular short breaks at work to stretch and use inactive muscles.
▶ Join a social dance group and spend as much time as you can on the dance floor.

## QUICK AND EASY EXERCISE STEPS

Tighten and tone your thighs and abdomen with these 4 easy, daily exercise steps.

### Inner and Outer Thighs
▶ Stand tall with your legs apart.
▶ Bend your knees, so they come directly above your feet.
▶ Now, lower your body, increasing the bend; hold this position for 4 counts.
▶ Slowly lift your body to its original position, and hold for a count of 4.
▶ Repeat until your legs start to tire. Gradually work up to doing 10 continuous repetitions each day.

### Upper Abdomen
▶ Lie flat on your back with your knees bent and your feet flat on the floor.
▶ Breathe in. As you breathe out, lift your head and chest, reaching forward with your hands towards your knees.
▶ Lower yourself gently to the floor.
▶ Repeat the whole exercise again until you tire. Work up to 10 continuous repetitions each day.
▶ Repeat the routine, reaching forward with your right hand to your left knee. Repeat, alternating from right hand to left hand, 10 times.

### Lower Abdomen
▶ Lie on your back, with your knees bent. Place your hands under your head.
▶ Bring your knees up and in towards your head, while reaching forward with your elbows to meet your knees. Repeat until you tire. Work up to 20 repeats. A slow, controlled movement is best.

### Bottom and Backs of Thighs
▶ Kneel on all fours, then place your elbows on the floor, leaving your bottom up.
▶ Push your right knee up behind you in a donkey kick, keeping your knee bent. Return to your original starting position.
▶ Repeat 5 times with your right leg, then repeat the exercise with your left leg. Gradually work up to 10 repeats with each leg.

# EXERCISE CHOICES

## WALKING

This is a popular, good all-round exercise choice for many people. It is convenient, requires no expensive equipment, and can be done by anyone of any age. Walk fast enough to cover about 6 kilometres in an hour. Step out in stride and swing your arms from side to side, ensuring that your torso, as well as your lower body, becomes involved in your exercising.

If you are overweight, sedentary or unfit, begin with short distances, and aim to increase the distance with each walk. Research has shown that you will use up the same number of kilojoules walking a set distance, whether you walk it in 20 minutes or 45 minutes.

## JOGGING

Many people like to jog or run as part — or all — of their exercise regime. Unlike walking, however, jogging or running can cause joint injury, sprained tendons or 'shin splints' (painful bruising of the calf). Jogging is also not for the very overweight or unfit.

If jogging or running is your exercise of choice, start out with brisk walks interspersed with jogging or running to build up stamina. A modest 3-kilometre run each day will keep your body in good condition, and, best of all, it can be accomplished in under ½ hour, which is a big plus for busy people.

Before you kick up a cloud of dust you should be aware of the following:

▶ You will need a good pair of running shoes, with plenty of support and cushioning. Ordinary sandshoes will not provide the necessary support.
▶ Try to jog or run on grass or soft dirt, as concrete causes high impact on your joints.
▶ Always begin with a 5 minute warm-up of stretching exercises.

▶ If you really want to jog but still have apprehensions about possible injury, bounce on a mini-trampoline. In fact this will give you all the benefits of running without the problems associated with injury or the weather.

## SWIMMING

This is by far the most refreshing and tension-draining form of exercise. Swimming works your whole body without overstraining your joints. It will tone many major muscles, as well as providing a good aerobic workout.

All strokes will improve your fitness level and burn up kilojoules. The most demanding and efficient strokes for this purpose, though, are freestyle and butterfly.

Start your swimming regime with 1 or 2 50-metre laps, followed by 2 minutes' rest, followed by more laps, repeating the process until you tire. As your stamina increases, so will your capacity to do laps, until you are swimming 20–30 continuous Olympic-length laps.

## CYCLING

As well as burning kilojoules, cycling offers one of the best cardiovascular workouts. For people who do not have the time to cycle around the countryside, consider buying a stationary exercise bike. You can achieve the same result — all you need is the self-discipline and motivation to ride it regularly.

If cycling is for you, aim to cruise at about 10 kilometres per hour on level ground, and don't use the easier gears too often.

## AEROBICS

Joining a health and fitness centre's exercise classes is a time-efficient way to ensure that you get your exercise. Start at a beginner's level to avoid muscle soreness, then progress through the various levels as you build up stamina. Vary your classes — low-impact aerobics, stretch-and-tone muscles, or circuit, interspersed with a minute's vigorous jogging to keep your heart rate up. And always follow the leader's instructions carefully — this will help you avoid injury.

## KILOJOULE BURNERS

Each category represents the number of kilojoules burned per minute when engaging in that form of exercise.

### LIGHT (10–20 KJ)
Walking, slow; lawn/tenpin bowling; golf; table tennis; housework, light; gardening, light; yoga; waterskiing; surfing.

### MODERATE (20–30 KJ)
Walking, fast; gardening, heavy; tennis; bicycling; horse riding; skating; swimming, moderate; ballroom dancing; hockey.

### HEAVY (30–40 KJ)
Jogging; skipping; dancing; climbing stairs; aerobics; downhill skiing; netball; football; sailing.

### VERY HEAVY (40 KJ AND OVER)
Swimming, training; squash, advanced; cross-country skiing; marathon running; rowing; basketball; uphill hiking; fast bicycling.

# Eyes

Eyes are the focal point of your face. These delicate mechanisms should be treated with respect, and any trouble should be referred immediately to an optician.

To keep your eyes clear and bright you need plenty of sleep and relaxation, as well as a good, mixed, healthy diet. If you lack sleep or have been overindulging in alcohol, eating rich foods or smoking, the appearance of your eyes will suffer. To avoid tired, strained and bloodshot eyes, make sure you take plenty of vitamin A (found in carrots and apricots), sleep for 8 hours a night as often as possible, and refrain from watching too much television.

It is also important not to read or use your eyes for close work in inadequate light. If you work on a computer, take a break every hour or so. And don't forget to blink — it cleanses and massages the eye. Bilberry, available from health food stores and chemists as a supplement, will help strengthen your eyes.

Whenever your eyes have been exposed to a smoky atmosphere, salt water, excessive wind and sun, or long hours working under artificial light, refresh them with a soothing herbal eyebath. To make your eye lotion, put 2 tablespoons of fresh parsley or 1 teaspoon of dried parsley in a ceramic bowl. Cover with 300 ml of boiling water, steep until the liquid becomes tepid, then strain through muslin or cheesecloth. Bathe your eyes as required, using an eyebath.

Distilled witch hazel (available from chemists) will also soothe and ease tired eyes, and help reduce puffiness. Moisten 2 cotton wool balls with the witch hazel, but don't let them become so wet that the liquid runs into your eyes, and place one over each eye. Lie back and relax for 15 minutes while the witch hazel does its job.

A quick and easy treatment to use when you're feeling tired and your eyelids feel heavy, is to lie down in a quiet, semi-darkened room with your eyes closed and your feet raised above the level of your head, and apply slices of cucumber to your eyelids. Tea bags are also effective — squeeze out excess moisture and put them on after they have cooled down. Thin slices of raw potato can be used for slight puffiness or a bruised sensation.

## DAY-TO-DAY EYE CARE

The skin under the eye is very thin and delicate, and care should be taken when removing make-up. Use a very fine oil, such as apricot or almond, to remove it, so that it floats off.

After cleansing, it is important to tone this tissue to ensure that the skin retains its elasticity. Gently pat distilled witch hazel onto the skin surrounding your eyes, avoiding an overgenerous application, as this will only cause stinging.

*See also Bilberry, Chamomile, Conjunctivitis.*

# F

## Fasting

Fasting is the most powerful of all tools for cleansing the body. It is necessary to help heal and eliminate diseases, growths, mucus, toxins and parasites.

The time to fast is when your body's natural capacity to eliminate toxins is impaired, or has become inefficient, and is interfering with the proper functioning of your body systems. When this happens, your body will send out obvious warnings:

- ▶ aches, pains, unclear head, frequent stomach upsets and menstrual cramps
- ▶ chronic constipation and associated tightness about the region of the shoulderblades
- ▶ black, offensive-smelling faecal matter
- ▶ offensive body odours
- ▶ inability to concentrate, dizziness and uncontrolled temper
- ▶ continuous tiredness — the feeling that you haven't had enough sleep, or need more sleep. A healthy body only requires from 2–6 hours' sleep, depending on whether you live in a natural, country setting or in the city
- ▶ insomnia
- ▶ lines on the face and that feeling 'I'm getting old', and lack of get-up-and-go
- ▶ dull or bloodshot eyes and sallow, ageing skin
- ▶ no appetite, eating from habit, and addiction to anything sweet, starches, coffee and cigarettes, overeating

- waking in the morning with an acid, bitter or salty taste in the mouth, a stuffy nose, mucus in the throat, encrustation in the eyes or wax in the ears
- coated tongue.

It is quite common for an individual to be congested with as much as 6.5 kg of extraneous mucus. As this is eliminated, more nutrients are able to reach the inner cells, thus improving the elimination of waste. Fasting is a natural, effective way for the body to rebuild its own dynamic healing powers.

There are a number of methods of fasting. You can eat only mild food, vegetable broth, fruit juices and water, or abstain from all food and water.

The latter is not recommended — nor is fasting over long periods (2 weeks or more) — without the supervision of a health practitioner. Avoid all supplementary vitamins and minerals, as they only interfere with the cleansing process. Drink herbal teas, though, as they will help cleanse your body and regulate your glands.

Most people tend to procrastinate when it comes to body housekeeping. Don't wait until you get sick before you commence regular fasting as part of your health programme.

Your body will react during your first fast. You may suffer symptoms including nausea, aching muscles, sleeplessness, headache, fatigue, irritability, a heavily coated tongue, loss of weight, foul breath and a sense of weakness. In rare instances, the reaction may include open sores, rashes and vomiting.

The first 3 days of a fast are the hardest, with the fast crisis usually occurring some time towards the end of the second day. By the third day you begin to feel the benefit, and you know the crisis is past when you feel extreme hunger. On each day of your fast you should:

- drink at least 8 glasses of liquid. This should be plain, distilled water, or water mixed with a little fresh fruit juice
- drink herbal teas

- have a cleansing enema — every evening for the first 3 days to clean filth from your colon
- have a dry brush massage
- have a hot and cold shower, or bath, to induce perspiration
- go for a walk or do some other exercise
- have at least one hour's rest during the day
- eat a vegetable broth — but only if you have to work during the fast, and if absolutely necessary. Otherwise, use a vegetable broth to break your fast.

## LIQUID FAST

A liquid fast is ideal for those fasting for the first time. It maintains a high energy level, thus allowing activity. A water fast, with no fruit juice, herbal tea, etc., is best for healthy people who have maintained a natural lifestyle over a number of years.

The fasting phase lasts for 3 days and breaking it lasts for 4 days — a week altogether. When breaking your fast, be careful not to stuff yourself with food. Not only will eating too much reduce the effect of the cleansing, it can also cause serious damage. It is important, when you eat straight after fasting, that all your food is at room temperature and in small portions. Practise this cleansing routine once every second month.

Day 1          Drink a minimum of 8 glasses of liquid —
               distilled water and fresh fruit juice, fruit juice
               cocktail (at least 4 glasses) and herbal tea. Drink
               vegetable broth, if you are working, but only
               2 glasses.

Days 2 and 3   Repeat as for Day 1. Remember — 4 glasses of
               fruit juice cocktail.

Day 4          One piece of fruit for breakfast. Light vegetable
               and sprout salad for lunch. Two glasses of fruit
               juice cocktail — one at lunch, the other for
               dinner. Six glasses of water.

| Day 5 | Repeat Day 4. Include 1 bowl of vegetable broth for the evening and have 2 extra pieces of fruit. |
|---|---|
| Day 6 | Increase your fruit intake. Add more vegetables and sprouts to the lunchtime salad. Add unsalted nuts to your diet. Dinner can consist of vegetable broth, bread and butter, and a small portion of baked vegetables. Drink one glass of fruit juice cocktail with each meal and before going to bed. |
| Day 7 | Recommence eating mild food. |

### *Fruit Juice Cocktail*

Use only fresh herbs and fruit.
*1 large pineapple, peeled and sliced*
*125 ml orange juice*
*1 handful parsley*
*2 stalks celery*

Process all the ingredients in a blender, and strain before drinking.
Makes 4 servings.

### *Vegetable Broth*

*2 large red potatoes (skins included)*
*3 stalks celery*
*3 medium beets*
*4 carrots*
*1/2 small head cabbage*
*3 onions*
*fresh basil, parsley and thyme*

Finely chop or grate all vegetables and add to a pot containing
1.5 litres of boiling water. Season with parsley, basil and thyme.
Cover and simmer for 45 minutes. When slightly cool, process in a
blender and drink warm.

# ENEMAS

Fasting uses the eliminative organs extensively to remove concentrated waste from your body. If your colon is congested, these toxins will be absorbed back into your body, causing sore throat, earache, fever, headache and numerous other illnesses. Therefore it is important to use an enema to clean out the colon.

A garlic and cayenne enema should be used each evening for the first 3 days of the fast.

To make an enema you will need three enema bags (available from most chemists), filled with distilled water. The first bag must be warm water to relax the colon; the second and third bags should be filled with slightly cool water, to stimulate the automatic muscular movement of the colon.

To use the enema bag, first lubricate the delivery tube with petroleum jelly and then insert it just inside the rectum. As the water starts to run in, gradually insert the tube further, but no more than 20 cm and only as long as it slides easily — never force it. Once you feel a cramp or the urge to expel, immediately remove the tube and relax for easy elimination. Do this for all 3 bags, then eat some fresh natural yogurt to replace the natural bacteria lost from the colon.

## GARLIC AND CAYENNE ENEMA

Do not use this if you have, or suspect that you have, any serious bowel problems.

Blend 2 cloves of garlic and ½ teaspoon of cayenne in 1 litre of water. Strain, and add sufficient water to fill a bag. Repeat for each bag.

# BODY BRUSH MASSAGE

The skin is the largest eliminative organ of the body. Dust, dirt, pollution and inactivity will cause its pores to become clogged and congested. Daily body brushing is essential, especially when you are fasting, to open the pores and allow the toxins to escape by increasing the flow of lymph. In addition, the skin is exfoliated, leaving it smooth, soft and glowing.

This simple procedure can be carried out for a few minutes each day, while you are taking a shower. Use only a body brush or loofah. If you don't have a loofah or body brush handy, you can exfoliate and brush your body by adding 2 tablespoons of medium oatmeal and 2 tablespoons of dried chamomile to a bath bag. Simply place the ingredients on a square of muslin, draw up the sides and tie with a ribbon.

A friction massage with a loofah or friction mitt during a warm bath is also good for accelerating cell metabolism and improving circulation. Coarse sea salt on the loofah helps improve skin colour, and is excellent for clearing flaking skin and spots. Always massage upwards, in the direction of the heart.

For stubborn areas on the lower legs and thighs, massage with coarse sea salt or an oatmeal bath bag, rinse off thoroughly, and pat dry with a towel. Then massage the legs with the following lotion, using rotating movements on the cellulite areas.

### *Leg Massage Oil*

*15 ml almond oil*
*2 drops jojoba oil*
*2 drops carrot oil*
*7 drops cypress essential oil*
*3 drops juniper essential oil*
*2 drops lavender essential oil*

Combine all the oils in a medicine glass or ceramic eggcup, mixing until thoroughly blended. Use the lotion generously, massaging it well into your skin. Maintain firm strokes, and keep massaging until all traces of the lotion have disappeared.

# PERSPIRATION

Perspiration is another important way the body naturally rids itself of toxins. A hot bath, which induces perspiration, should be taken regularly to induce perspiration as part of your cleansing regime. During fasting, if you include certain herbs in the bathwater, perspiration will open your pores and increase your circulation.

### Cleansing Bath Herbs

*1 cup cider vinegar*
*½ cup salt*
*3 tablespoons ground ginger*

Mix these together and add to warm bathwater. Remain in the tub until perspiration ceases, and sip several glasses of water while you're there. Drinking water will help eliminate toxins faster.
When perspiration ceases, immediately take a cold shower to close your skin pores.

It is quite common for people to suffer dizziness when sitting in a hot bath for a prolonged period. Prevent this by providing plenty of ventilation: open windows and doors, use a fan to circulate air and place a cool cloth across your forehead.

If you have a fever, do not take a hot bath. Instead, have a cold bath, with the same herbs included, to help bring the fever down.

---

**Warning:** *People with heart or blood pressure problems are easily affected by sudden temperature changes from hot to cold. This is a definite risk to those over 50 who are predisposed to arteriosclerosis, or who have a poorly functioning heart. Such a decline in blood pressure could be the catalyst for a mild stroke.*

*See also Bathing.*

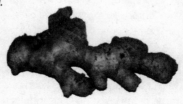

## EXERCISE

Blocked circulation is the main cause of illness; regular exercise is important, because it increases your circulation. It will help toxins move through your lymphatic system, and remove them through your eliminative organs.

Usually exercise is needed most when you least feel like doing it. It should be part of your fasting routine, and in your daily health programme.

Long, brisk walks are excellent (not jogging, since this can cause damage to the organs and skeletal system), as is jumping up and down on a mini-trampoline.

*See also Water.*

## FRESH AIR

Fresh air and being outdoors also help maintain good health. However, make sure you cover up, as it is important to protect yourself from the sun's damaging rays.

## WATER

*See Water.*
*See also Herbal Detox.*

# Fatigue

It is not uncommon to feel a little fatigued and out of sorts from time to time. An inadequate and improper diet — in particular, insufficient intake of vitamins and minerals — is usually the cause of this condition. Lack of B group vitamins, especially vitamin B12, and the mineral magnesium can cause chronic irritability, exhaustion and mental fatigue.

Although supplements are readily available, it is far better to maintain a well-balanced diet that includes fresh fruit and vegetables and plenty of herbs. Foods to help motivate you and get you going are apples, bananas, corn, grapefruit, mangoes, pawpaw, peaches and yellow squash. A small glass of fresh carrot juice each day is also an excellent boost for your system — of all the juices, it has the best balance of vitamins and minerals.

Natural food sources of magnesium are almonds and other nuts, fish, prawns, leafy green vegetables, molasses, soya beans, sunflower seeds and wheat germ. Herbs which provide this element are alfalfa (eat daily as sprouted seed), cayenne, dandelion and peppermint. Fresh dandelion leaves can be cooked like spinach; the young, tender leaves can be chopped up and served in a salad.

B group vitamin food sources are brewer's yeast (sprinkle over breakfast cereal), grains and seeds (such as wheat germ), rice bran, sunflower seeds, nuts, legumes, potatoes, almonds, mushrooms, soya beans, citrus fruits, molasses, spinach, cauliflower, salmon and some dairy products. Vitamin B12 can be found in most meats; remember, meat should be lean and eaten sparingly. Herb sources of B complex vitamins are dandelion, fenugreek, parsley, alfalfa, watercress, cayenne, burdock and sage.

If you're feeling tired and in need of a quick energy fix, try a banana. Mashed and mixed with a little honey and avocado, and served on oat biscuits, it makes a powerful energy-packed snack.

For a good start to the day, kick off with the following energy-packed breakfast. Soak 1 handful each of sultanas and raisins overnight and reserve the soakwater. Mix together the sultanas and raisins, including the soakwater, 2 handfuls of sprouted wheat, 1 piece of apple, finely chopped, 1 tablespoon of fresh yogurt, 1 piece of finely diced seasonal fruit, and 1 handful of ground mixed nuts. Sprinkle with a pinch of powdered cinnamon and powdered vanilla bean.

Most importantly, though, when you are feeling tired, irritable and exhausted, first assess what you are eating; if necessary, change your diet to include plenty of fresh fruit and vegetables and herbs. This will give you the energy to get out and continue to enjoy life, rather than sleeping it away.

## ENERGY-PACKED FRUIT SALAD

A great way to boost energy levels during the day. Use any or all of the following fresh fruits, if available: 1 small pineapple, diced; 2 peaches, sliced; 2 medium mangoes, sliced; 2 pears, diced; 2 oranges, diced; 1 apple, diced; 375 g ricotta cheese, crumbled.

Place the prepared fruit in a bowl. Add the cheese and stir slightly until the fruit is evenly distributed, then chill and serve. As a lunch meal this is complete in itself, supplying abundant protein, vitamins and minerals.

## EXERCISE

A brisk 20–30 minute walk (not a jog, as this can cause damage to your organs and skeletal system) is a great feel-good activity because it gives you energy. Do this at least 3 times a week, either first thing in the morning or after dinner at night, but no later than 2 hours before bed. Walk at a pace that's fast enough to allow you to cover about 6 kilometres in an hour. Stride out and swing your arms from side to side, thus ensuring that your torso, and not just your lower body, becomes involved.

*See also Exercise.*

## ESSENTIAL OILS

An aromatic shower, using essential oils, is a great way to start the day and boost your energy levels. Invigorating and energising oils include clary sage, rosemary, tangerine, orange, lime and lemon grass.

*To take advantage of essential oils in your morning shower, see Aromatic Shower.*

*See also Dietary Substitutes, Eating for Health and Energy, Exercise, Massage, Mental Fatigue, Revitalisation, Stress and Tension.*

# Feet

Feet are often the most neglected part of our body, yet within the average lifetime they will walk the equivalent of 4 times around the world. Tired feet make for a tired-looking face, so take the time to give your feet the attention and care they deserve.

At the end of a busy day, a therapeutic footbath and a quick massage will work wonders for tired and aching feet. Soaking your feet in a footbath at night before going to bed will help eliminate lots of toxins.

Before soaking your feet, give each one a preliminary massage. Prepare your foot massage oil by thoroughly mixing together 15 ml of almond oil, 5 ml of avocado oil and 6 drops of rosemary essential oil. Store in an airtight, amber-coloured glass bottle for up to 2 months.

Pour a little oil into your hands and hold your left foot firmly. Press along the underneath area and the upper surface for about 20 seconds. This will induce a marvellous feeling of relaxation.

Next, place your left foot over your knee. Press, rub and pull each toe, and knead the sole with your knuckles. Then place the fingers of both hands on the sole, and the thumbs, pointing toward the toes, on top of your foot. Stroke down from the ankles to the toes. Repeat this whole procedure with your other foot.

To soak your feet, you will need a basin large enough to hold them when they are fully stretched out. Pour in enough water to cover your ankles and then add 1 tablespoon of sea salt or Epsom salts and 3–4 drops of lavender or rosemary essential oil. Swish the water around to dissolve the salt and blend the oil. For extra-sore and aching feet add 1 tablespoon each of sea salt and bicarbonate of soda and 3–5 drops of rosemary essential oil to the water.

Leave the water to cool slightly before soaking your feet. After soaking them for 10 minutes, revive your feet with a quick dip into a basin of cold water, then return them to the footbath. Continue doing this as long as the water in the footbath stays hot.

If it has been raining and you have cold, wet feet, a pinch or two of mustard powder added to the water is especially invigorating.

Finish off by massaging your feet with a soothing herbal lotion made by blending together 6 drops of rosemary oil, 15 ml of almond oil and 5 ml of avocado oil. Store any remaining lotion in a small, amber-coloured glass bottle in a cool, dark cupboard.

If you don't have the time for a separate footbath, rub rosemary essential oil or diluted apple cider vinegar into your feet, massaging for about 5 minutes, before you take a bath.

## PEOPLE IN A HURRY

If you are in a hurry, a quick soak in a basin of water to which has been added a few drops of peppermint essential oil will soon perk you up. It is extremely refreshing, and marvellous after a long day on your feet.

## PEOPLE WHO ENJOY WALKING

For those of you who enjoy a lot of walking, give your feet a quick soak in a footbath using geranium (pelargonium) essential oil before you set out. It strengthens your skin, improves elasticity and circulation, and helps prevent blisters.

## DRY SKIN

If you suffer from dry skin on your feet, wash them with a mixture of 1 tablespoon of bran and 3 tablespoons of strong chamomile tea (about 3 level teaspoons of dried chamomile steeped in 300 ml of hot water until cold). Rinse, wipe dry, and then moisturise with your favourite hand cream or lotion.

## HARD SKIN

Soften very hard skin on the soles of your feet or the backs of your heels by massaging with equal quantities of olive oil and cider vinegar. Smooth daily with a natural pumice stone.

## QUICK AND SIMPLE FOOT EXERCISE

This simple and quick foot exercise will help your feet recover from the confinement of shoes. Gently stretch the arch of each foot and curl your toes underneath. Hold this position and count to 10. Do this 3 times with each foot whenever you are sitting down.

## FOOT CARE GUIDELINES

Most foot problems are caused by a lack of care and badly fitting shoes. This can be avoided by following a few simple guidelines.

▶ Let your feet breathe — walk barefoot as often as possible to let your feet recover from the confinement of shoes.

▶ Wear sensible footwear — flat-heeled, comfortable leather shoes or sandals — whenever possible.

▶ Shop for shoes in the afternoon, as your feet swell during the day. And make sure that shoes are at least 2.5 cm longer than your feet.

▶ Avoid wearing the same pair of shoes every day, and avoid buying plastic shoes; choose leather or fabric which will allow your feet to breathe.

▶ Wear socks made from natural fibres because they breathe; synthetics will encourage perspiration.

▶ Sprinkle a little dry, powdered chamomile (reduce the chamomile to a powder by rubbing it through a fine wire sieve) mixed with an equal amount of bicarbonate of soda into shoes after wearing them for the whole day.

▶ At the end of a busy day, give your feet a soothing massage and footbath.

▶ Prevent foot odour and excessive perspiration by including sufficient silica in your diet; eat barley, garlic, onion, parsley, lettuce and celery. Bathe your feet in a bowl of hot water containing a few drops of lemon grass oil, then apply a lotion made by combining 18 drops of lemon grass oil and 30 ml of soya oil. Store the mixture in an airtight, amber-coloured glass bottle.

*See also Athlete's Foot, Foot Odour, Thyme.*

# Feverfew

Feverfew (*Tanacetum parthenium*) is a common, rather fragrant member of the daisy family that was known to the ancient Egyptians and Greeks, who regarded it as a valuable remedy for alleviating headaches, joint pain, stomach aches and fever. Today researchers have confirmed that feverfew is a valuable herbal remedy that is especially effective in treating migraine headaches and arthritis, and some types of menstrual problems.

Feverfew contains a number of lactones, among them parthenolide, michefuscalide and chrysanthenyl. The main active sesquiterpene lactone, parthenolide, is known to inhibit the production and secretion of prostaglandins, substances released by blood platelets and white blood cells that contribute to migraines. White blood cells also secrete substances believed to contribute to the kind of inflammatory processes seen in arthritis and possibly some other auto-immune disorders. Another substance, serotonin, is also secreted by blood platelets and can constrict blood vessels and contribute to migraine pain. This inhibition of prostaglandins results in reduction in inflammation, decreased secretion of histamine, and a reduction of fevers, thus the name feverfew.

Apart from its general tonic abilities, feverfew can be taken as a preventive for migraine headaches.

*See Headaches, Migraine Headaches.*

# Fibre in Your Diet

*See Nutrition, Fibre.*

# Fingernails

*See Hand Care.*

# First Aid

*See Medicinal Oils, Tea-Tree Oil.*

# Fish Oils

*See Cod Liver Oil.*

# Flatulence

We all suffer from flatulence from time to time. This common problem is usually due to overeating, eating too rapidly, or eating unsuitable, hard-to-digest foods. If the problem persists and is causing you distress, you should seek professional advice. However, in most circumstances it can be dispelled and eased by the use of herbs.

The principal herbs for dispelling gas from the stomach and bowels are allspice, aniseed, caraway seed, cloves, sweet fennel, ginger, peppermint, thyme and parsley. Drink any of these herbs as a hot herbal tea whenever you suffer from wind in the stomach or intestines.

To make your herbal tea, place 1 teaspoon of dried ground herb in a ceramic cup, add boiling water, cover and steep for 3 minutes. Strain into another cup and reheat if necessary.

A dose of ¼ teaspoon of powdered angelica root is also a very gentle way to quickly expel gas from the stomach and bowel. It is safe to be taken by children.

Wind associated with colic pain, due to distension of the intestinal walls, should be treated as follows: mix together ½ teaspoon each of ground aniseed, ground dried peppermint and ground fennel seed. Add the mixture to 500 ml of water and boil for 5 minutes.

98

Drink 1 cup of the brew while it is still hot. If the pain persists after 15–20 minutes, drink another cup of tea.

Unless the pain is a result of a very serious obstruction, it will ease in 10–30 minutes. If it does not, seek professional help.

*See also Herbal Teas, Indigestion, Medicinal Food.*

# Floral Vinegar

For many centuries aromatic vinegars were used to ward off infections. You can use them as a refreshing and invigorating addition to a hot bath, as an astringent and skin softener, to relieve headaches and to soothe a throbbing temple after exposure to the sun. They can also be made into a cooling wash to clean the face or a skin toner to be used after cleansing. Floral vinegar also does wonders to freshen up a sickroom.

Their refreshing and healing quality is due to acetic acid, which dissolves the aromatic and other beneficial substances found in herbs and flower petals.

Floral vinegars are best made with a good-quality cider vinegar, which can be infused with herbs such as rose petals, lavender, rosemary, lemon balm, lemon verbena, basil, hyssop, peppermint, scented geranium leaves and jasmine.

To make your floral vinegar, half fill a clear wide-mouthed glass jar with fresh chopped herbs and top up with warmed vinegar. Seal the jar and leave it for 3–4 weeks in a spot where it will receive plenty of sunlight. Strain off the vinegar, squeezing all liquid from the herbs, and then dilute it by adding an equal amount of distilled water.

If you find it more convenient to use dried herbs or petals to make a floral vinegar, put 3 tablespoons of herbs or 6 tablespoons of petals in a ceramic bowl. Mix together 300 ml each of good-quality cider vinegar and distilled water, and heat to just below boiling point. Pour the liquid over the herbs, cover tightly with plastic wrap and leave to steep for 12 hours. Strain and bottle for future use.

## IN THE BATH

Use your floral vinegar in the bathroom by adding 1 cup of your chosen vinegar to the bath while the taps are running, or soak a soft face cloth in the vinegar, then wring it out and lay it across your forehead while you relax.

## FACIAL SKIN CARE

For washing your face, mix 2 tablespoons of lavender vinegar with 1 cup of rosewater (available from most chemists and health food stores) and store in an airtight glass bottle. Apply directly to the face, then rinse off. If lavender isn't the herb of choice for your skin type, use a more suitable herb to create your own astringent vinegar face wash. Basil and lemon verbena is suitable for oily and disturbed skins, jasmine works well on sensitive skin, and violet petals or scented geranium leaves (*Pelargonium* spp.) will suit all skin types.

To make a toner, to use on your skin after cleansing or removing make-up, dilute 20 ml of floral vinegar with 150 ml of distilled water and store in a glass bottle. Pour a little of the toner onto slightly damp cotton wool, and gently apply to your face and neck, using outward and upward movements.

## HEADACHE

Whenever headache from stress or strain persists, dampen a handkerchief with lavender vinegar and lay it across your forehead for 5–10 minutes.

---

*See also Headache, Stress and Tension.*

## SICKROOM

Floral vinegars can also be used to make the surroundings more pleasant for someone confined to bed. Simply soak a small sponge in lavender vinegar and leave it in a dish beside the bed. Renew the lavender vinegar as needed.

## SUN EXPOSURE

After exposure to the hot sun, dab lavender, rose or lemon verbena vinegar behind your ears and on your temples and forehead.

*See also Sunstroke.*

# Folate

Folate is a B vitamin found in a variety of foods and added to many vitamin and mineral supplements as folic acid, a synthetic form of folate. Folate is needed both before and in the first weeks of pregnancy and can help reduce the risk of serious and common birth defects called neural tube defects, which affect the brain and spinal cord.

Folate occurs naturally in a variety of foods, primarily in dark green leafy vegetables, but also in beneficial quantities in asparagus, broccoli, citrus fruits and juices and mushrooms; in oysters, salmon, strawberries, whole-grain products, wheat germ and yeast; and dried beans and peas, such as lima, navy and soya beans, and chickpeas. Some breakfast cereals (ready-to-eat and others) are fortified with folic acid.

A deficiency of folate can occur when your need for folate is increased, when dietary intake of folate is inadequate, and when your body excretes (or loses) more folate than usual. Some situations that increase the need for folate include pregnancy and lactation (breastfeeding), alcohol abuse, kidney dialysis and liver disease.

Signs of folic acid deficiency are usually subtle, and are associated with symptoms such as diarrhoea, loss of appetite and weight loss. Additional indicators can be a general feeling of weakness, sore tongue, headaches, heart palpitations, irritability and behavioural disorders.

Women with folate deficiency who become pregnant are more likely to give birth to low birth weight and premature infants, and infants with neural tube defects.

In adults, anaemia is a sign of advanced folate deficiency. In infants and children, folate deficiency can slow growth rate. Some of these symptoms can also result from a variety of medical conditions other than folate deficiency. It is important to have a health practitioner evaluate these symptoms so that appropriate medical care can be given.

# Folic Acid

*See Folate, Eating for Health and Energy (Broccoli, Spirulina).*

# Food Poisoning

Food poisoning can be caused by bacteria, carried by humans or flies, or rotten food. Symptoms usually occur within 48 hours of eating the offending meal. Diarrhoea is the most likely effect, and often accompanied by nausea, pain and vomiting.

Castor oil is one of the best remedies for food poisoning. Take 2 tablespoons of castor oil when symptoms are evident. Also, drink plenty of fluids and get some bed rest.

# Foot Odour

*See Feet.*

# Fungal Problems

*See Athlete's Foot, Thyme.*

# G

## Gallstones

You should seek expert medical advice if you suspect you have this painful and distressing complaint. Symptoms are colic in the liver region, with a radiating pain to the back and right shoulder which is worse when the stomach is empty.

The inclusion of olive oil, with its strong lubricating properties, in the diet helps prevent gallstones. Dandelion tea is a very effective natural diuretic: take it as a tea, or include fresh young leaves in salads.

My grandmother, who was an old-time herbalist, left me a wealth of remedies and treatments. The following treatment for gallstones was found among the mountains of paper that I inherited from her.

*Dissolve 1 teaspoon of Epsom salts in water and drink it.*
*Forty-five minutes later swallow a good mouthful of olive oil,*
*immediately followed by a mouthful of lemon juice and again another*
*good mouthful of olive oil. Lie down on your left side for approximately*
*20 minutes. Repeat the procedure twice more.*

## Garlic (*Allium astirum*)

Garlic is considered to be a natural antibiotic if taken in large enough doses. It contains vitamins A, B and C, copper, sulphur, manganese, iron and calcium, and because its oil is composed of sulphides and disulphides, garlic inactivates undesirable virulent micro-organisms in the body, without harming the helpful organisms.

When winter is just around the corner it's important to build up your body's resistance to infection. And what better and more natural way to do this than to use garlic to help boost your body's defences.

It helps prevent colds and expel catarrh from the chest, acts as an antiseptic, will soothe a nagging cough, and relieves the symptoms of sinusitis.

If you take garlic on a regular basis it will cleanse cholesterol and toxins from your bloodstream, aid your digestion, cleanse stale mucus from your tissues, nourish your nerves and increase your glandular secretions.

However, you must be mindful of the fact that no matter how you take fresh garlic, after a while your body fragrance will be astounding. If others around you find this offensive, you can buy odourless garlic tablets from health food stores.

To sweeten the breath after taking fresh garlic, eat a sprig of parsley.

Used as an enema or internally it will kill various kinds of worms and parasites. In cases of yeast infection use garlic water as a douche; for babies, wash the affected area.

Made into an ointment, it is said to relieve rheumatic pain and muscular strain.

## GARLIC COLD CURE

The following drink is ideal for people who do not take garlic on a regular basis and begin to suffer the symptoms of a cold, or have a bad cold.

*2 cloves crushed garlic*
*½ teaspoon ground ginger*
*1 tablespoon honey*
*juice of 1 lemon*
*pinch cayenne pepper*
*1 cup boiling water*

Put all the ingredients in a prewarmed ceramic cup. Add the boiling water, cover and allow to steep for 10 minutes. Strain, reheat and drink immediately.

# GARLIC OINTMENT

Use for muscular strains and rheumatic pain.

*2 cloves garlic*
*100 g petroleum jelly*

Crush the cloves and mix well with the petroleum jelly. Store in
an airtight jar.
Rub well into the affected area when required.

# GARLIC SOUP

The more red meat you eat, the more you need a
good amino acid balance. Although red meat does
contain these acids, the digestive tract may not be
in a clean enough state to adequately cope with the
digestion and easy assimilation of protein. This causes
stomach rumblings and offensive antisocial gases.

To avoid this problem it is important to include
natural sources of sulphur in your diet — avocados,
celery, cucumber, mushrooms, tomatoes, onions
(all types) and garlic.

Garlic is especially useful for cleansing
toxins from your bloodstream, as well as
aiding in digestion and cleansing stale mucus from
your tissues. In my family, the favourite way of
enjoying and taking advantage of the many benefits
of garlic is by eating my grandmother's garlic soup.

*8 cloves of fresh garlic*
*2 large new potatoes, skins on*
*(Pontiacs are best if you can get them)*
*3–4 cups of water*
*1 bay leaf*
*a few sprigs fresh sage, chopped finely*
*a few sprigs fresh thyme, chopped finely*
*salt substitute (see Salt Substitute)*
*freshly ground black pepper*

Peel the garlic cloves and put them in a covered saucepan with the potatoes, cut into small chunks. Add water and bay leaf, then bring to the boil. Reduce heat and allow to simmer for 15 minutes. Cool, then add herbs and pepper. Sieve or blend the soup. Season and reheat to serve. The flavour of this soup increases the day after it is made. Although the flavour can't be compared, dried herbs can be substituted for fresh ones.

*See also Antibiotics, Nappy Rash, Yeast Infection.*

# Gastritis

I have found the following treatment to be very effective. Cut out all food, then take 1 tablespoon of castor oil in a glass of warm milk morning and night until the condition clears itself.

In cases where there is sudden and severe pain, slippery elm powder (available from health food stores) can be taken as an emergency treatment. As soon as you are aware of the pain, mix 1 tablespoon of the powder with a little fruit juice and take it. Take it once a day for a week.

# Gastro-intestinal Disorders

*See Acidity, Chamomile (Chamomile Tea), Gastritis, Herbal Teas (Lemon Balm), Indigestion, Overindulgence, Stomach.*

# Gentian

An extremely bitter-tasting herb, gentian (*Gentian lutea*) does improve the digestion of fats and protein. Included in a digestive tonic it will also alleviate digestive disturbances such as flatulence, constipation, heartburn, diarrhoea and nausea. It acts by stimulating the flow of gastric, liver and pancreatic digestive juices.

You can purchase liquid tonics containing gentian from health food stores.

# Ginseng

Ginseng (*Panax ginseng*) has been acclaimed as the herb of life in the annals of Chinese medicine for than 2000 years. It helps the body adapt more readily to physical and emotional stresses by strengthening the endocrine glands, the functions of which include the metabolism of vitamins and minerals, and builds vitality and resistance. Ginseng contains steroids similar to oestrogen, and when used in combination with sarsaparilla is reputed to help regulate the male hormones. Because it is a stimulant, you should reduce your intake of other stimulants, such as coffee, when you are taking ginseng.

You can buy ginseng as a whole root, in powder form, or as capsules, tablets or liquid extract, from health food stores.

# Glands

Swollen glands are usually the result of infection. The swelling can be reduced by aiding the movement of lymph; applying a compress to the affected area will do this. Dip a clean cloth in cider vinegar, squeeze it gently until it stops dripping, and apply it to the affected area. Keep it warm and covered. Renew as required.

Maintaining a regular daily exercise programme also helps. Exercise is one of the most important things that can be done to aid the movement of lymph through the body.

To prevent gland problems, your diet should include a generous intake of vitamin C, plus apples, pears, melons, oats and broccoli.

# Gout

Gout is caused by excessive uric acid build-up. The symptoms are usually severe inflammation around the big toes, but gout can occur in other joints. Include celery, carrots, cucumbers, cabbage, cauliflower, lettuce, tomatoes, freshly grated raw beetroot and mushrooms, parsley, fresh young nettle leaves (chopped raw in salads or lightly steamed), and grapes and strawberries in your diet.

Drink a cup of parsley, rosemary or sage tea twice a day. Add a pinch of cayenne to speed up the beneficial effect.

To relieve the discomfort of gout, apply a compress soaked in a strong infusion of sage. Use 2 tablespoons of dried herb in 300 ml of boiling water.

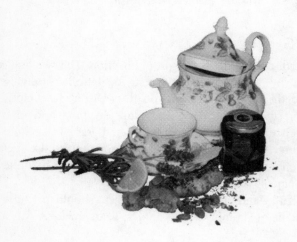

# Gums

*See Mouth.*

# H

## Haemorrhoids

Haemorrhoids, commonly called piles, are varicose veins of the rectal wall. They can be extremely painful and they often bleed a lot.

Include sweet potatoes, bananas, beans, plums, sweet corn, prunes and pumpkin in your diet, as well as plenty of roughage, such as psyllium-type products like Metamucil, which is available from chemists and supermarkets. Make sure you drink plenty of water when you take psyllium.

Splash cold water on your anus to help contract the haemorrhoids, and liberally apply borage ointment (*see Borage Ointment*). If necessary, wear a protective pad to prevent staining of undergarments and clothing. While applying the ointment, try to push any protruding haemorrhoids back up the rectal passage, but only if it can be done with ease.

Slippery elm powder will also give relief, especially if the problem is accompanied by constipation. Mix a tablespoonful of powder with a little water that has just been boiled to form a paste. Take twice a day. If you don't like the taste, mix in a little honey for a sweet, woody flavour. Because slippery elm is a mucilage herb, be sure to drink plenty of water each day when you are taking it.

Dandelion is excellent for treating piles and constipation. The leaf can be taken as a tea, or the root as a coffee substitute. Both dandelion tea and coffee are available from health food stores.

## Hair

Sun, wind and other climatic conditions can leave hair looking lifeless and dry. Even air pollution levels can contribute to unhealthy hair. The condition of your hair is also a fairly good indication of your general state of health.

A healthy balanced diet is a must; your hair needs vitamin B complex, vitamin A, calcium, silica, iron, zinc, protein and unsaturated oils or fatty acids. Eat plenty of fresh fruit, vegetables and salads, drink lots of water and make sure that you get enough sleep — 8 hours' rest each night will do wonders for your hair.

Although diet is the foundation of healthy hair, herbs will also help give it a natural, healthy appearance. Their gentle cleansing and conditioning action will leave your hair shiny and manageable. Those old-fashioned tips from great-grandma's day, like shampooing with an egg to bring life to dry hair and using lemon juice or vinegar rinse for oily hair, still work. Similarly, a traditional rosemary rinse after shampooing will help revitalise your scalp.

To make your rosemary hair lotion put 6 fresh, leafy sprigs of the herb (or 2 heaped tablespoons of the dried herb) in an enamel or stainless steel saucepan, add 5 cups of water and bring to the boil. Reduce heat and simmer for 15 minutes, keeping the lid on so that the vapour does not escape. Remove from heat, steep until cold and strain through muslin or cheesecloth.

Use as a final rinse after thoroughly rinsing out all traces of shampoo and conditioner. Massage well into your scalp with your fingertips. For sun-damaged hair replace the rosemary with 2 tablespoons each of dried chamomile and dried rosemary.

After swimming in salt or chlorinated water, wash your hair with a gentle, natural shampoo and then rinse with the rosemary lotion. You should also apply a herbal conditioner to your hair before you go swimming. As you swim it will slowly rinse away, protecting your hair from the harshness of chlorine or salt water.

## SCALP MASSAGE

A scalp massage will help keep your hair in better condition. Each evening before going to bed, press your fingertips against your scalp and rotate the skin underneath them gently.

# NOURISHING AND MOISTURISING YOUR SCALP

Your scalp can dry out just like your facial skin, leaving you with flaky skin and dandruff. This condition can be remedied by the regular use of a mildly antiseptic pre-wash conditioner that will stimulate, purify, nourish and moisturise your scalp.

This pre-wash conditioner has a base of almond oil, which is similar to your own scalp oil. It acts as an emollient, protecting your skin by replacing natural surface oils and preventing roughness and chapping.

*80 ml almond oil*
*10 ml avocado oil*
*10 ml wheat germ oil*
*1 drop peppermint essential oil*
*4 drops rosemary essential oil*

Thoroughly blend all the oils and store in an airtight, amber-coloured glass bottle away from heat. Use within 4 months.
Massage this conditioner into your scalp whenever it needs extra conditioning and dry flaky skin is evident.

# SHAMPOO

Since there is so much variation in hair type, colour and texture, it is important to use the correct shampoo for your individual needs. Choose from any of the herbs, singly or in combination, specified for your particular hair type (*see next page*).

*30 ml almond oil*
*30 ml castor oil*
*180 ml herbal infusion*
*6 drops essential oil/s of choice*

Combine all the ingredients in a suitable bottle, shake well, and store for future use. Shake before using. Massage into your wet scalp and hair for 1–2 minutes, then rinse thoroughly.

## HERBAL INFUSION

Prepare the infusion by adding 2 teaspoons of dried herbs (chosen from the shampoo herbs list below) to a ceramic bowl and covering with 300 ml of boiling water. Cover the bowl, steep until cold, strain through muslin cloth, and add the required amount to the base recipe.

For a stronger infusion, steep for 12 hours before straining.

## SHAMPOO HERBS

Choose from the following herbs according to your hair type. Prepare as directed for the herbal infusion.

### FAIR HAIR
Chamomile — has a lightening effect and helps scalp irritations.

### DARK HAIR
Rosemary or sage.

### DANDRUFF
Nettle, parsley, peppermint, rosemary or thyme. Thyme, rosemary and peppermint combined not only control dandruff but act as a scalp and hair tonic.

### OILY HAIR
Sage, yarrow, rosemary or lime (linden) flowers.

### HEALING
Chamomile, parsley, rosemary or peppermint.

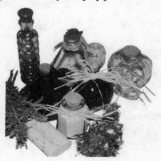

# MONTHLY PROTEIN CONDITIONER

This quick and easy-to-make protein conditioner can be applied to your hair once a month. It will keep your hair shiny and healthy, giving it life and bounce that everyone notices.

*20 ml almond oil*
*20 ml wheat germ oil*
*2 drops rosemary essential oil*
*1 drop lavender essential oil*
*20 ml glycerine*
*10 ml cider vinegar*
*1 egg*

Blend all the oils with the glycerine, add the vinegar, then beat well with the egg. After shampooing, massage the mixture thoroughly into your hair, cover with a shower cap and leave for 30 minutes. Shampoo out, rinse with clean water and then apply a herbal after-shampoo rinse.

# FALLING HAIR

This can result from illness, becoming run-down or a major hormonal upset. We all shed hair every day of our lives. Whenever you comb or brush, you lose some hair. However, when you start to notice that more hair is coming away in your hairbrush than normal, it is time to treat your hair.

Falling hair is not as serious as hair loss and you may find that a course of brewer's yeast tablets is all that is needed. Also, check your diet. Include plenty of fresh fruit and vegetables, cut down on stimulants such as coffee, tea and alcohol, and drink plenty of fresh water. Check your hair care habits: do not use chemical-based colorants, dyes and perms, and do not use hair dryers or other heat treatments excessively.

Use any of the shampoo herbs applicable to your hair type in the previous shampoo recipe, then add a beaten egg to a small amount of the mixture each time you wash your hair. Do not use hot water or the egg will scramble. Leave the shampoo on for as long as possible before you rinse it out.

Include a weekly treatment of the 'Monthly Protein Conditioner' after you have shampooed and rinsed out.

*See also Dandruff, Nettle, Sage.*

# Hand Care

Our hands can suffer from the rigours of day-to-day living. They're affected by wind, sun, hot and cold weather, harsh cleaning agents and the many tasks they are required to perform daily. This causes the skin to become dry and scaly, or in severe cases, chapped and split.

As well as taking advantage of the natural protection offered by herbal softeners and moisturisers, keep your hands in top condition by following these golden rules:

▶ Always apply a protective barrier cream before commencing rough work, dishwashing or messy household jobs.

▶ Wear protective gloves for gardening and other household chores as often as possible.

▶ Avoid direct contact with chemical cleansers, or, better still, use only products that are kind to your skin.

▶ Moisturise your hands morning and night, and immediately after any rough work or contact with water.

▶ Clean ingrained dirt and stains from your hands by dipping them in warm almond oil, then rubbing them with a mixture of coarse sea salt and equal amounts of dried chamomile, sage and yarrow — enough to form a paste. This mixture is great for cleaning hands after a session in the garden.

▶ Keep a small bowl of fine bran near the kitchen sink or laundry tub. Instead of using soap, which can be very drying if used too often, dip your hands in the bran and rub thoroughly to cleanse them, then rinse off.

▶ If your hands are very dry, soak them for $\frac{1}{2}$ hour in warm almond oil with 2 drops of carrot oil added.

- Strengthen your fingernails by soaking them in a bowl of water to which 1 tablespoon of cider vinegar has been added.
- Clean stains from your fingernails by applying lemon juice with a small paintbrush twice a day.

## HAND-FRIENDLY ESSENTIAL OILS

Soak your hands for 10 minutes each day in a bowl of warm water to which healing or therapeutic oils have been added. Add 2–4 drops of any of the following oils to a basin of warm water.

### DRY HANDS
Use rose, geranium or carrot.

### NEGLECTED HANDS
Use rose, geranium or lemon.

After soaking, massage in a generous amount of hand lotion made of equal quantities of lemon juice, glycerine and rosewater, not forgetting to include your wrists. Store remaining lotion in an airtight, amber-coloured glass bottle.

## PROTECTIVE HAND CREAM

This natural barrier cream will protect your hands from rough work, drying detergents and grime, and will help prevent your skin cracking and splitting.

Smooth it into your hands before you do any gardening or washing-up.

*25 g anhydrous lanolin*
*10 g beeswax*
*75 ml almond oil*
*40 ml lemon grass infusion*
*2 teaspoons lemon juice*
*3 drops friar's balsam (available from chemists)*

Prepare the infusion by adding a handful of the lemon grass to a ceramic bowl and just covering it with boiling water. Steep for 2 hours and strain.

Melt the lanolin and beeswax in a double boiler over medium heat. When liquid, add the almond oil and lemon grass infusion, stirring until well blended. Remove from heat, allow to cool, add lemon juice and friar's balsam and beat until cold and creamy.
Store in a sterilised glass jar with a tight-fitting lid.

## TOMATO HAND LOTION

Mix equal parts of tomato juice, lemon juice and glycerine. Massage well into your hands and wrists. This will cleanse as well as soften your skin.

## HONEY AND ALMOND NIGHT OIL

A rich, oily overnight conditioner for hands that have been excessively exposed to harsh climatic conditions. Massage well into your hands, then wear cotton gloves for increased absorption.

*1 teaspoon honey*
*1 tablespoon almond oil*
*1 tablespoon olive oil*
*2 teaspoons glycerine*

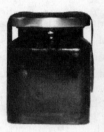

Gently warm the honey and oils in a double boiler until they are well blended. Remove from heat and beat in the glycerine.
Bottle and seal.

# FINGERNAILS

Many men and women suffer from brittle fingernails. Usually this type of problem indicates a dietary deficiency.

Most people know that calcium is necessary for strong nails, but few realise that the mineral silica is equally important. Foods that contain this mineral include barley, kelp, garlic, onions, parsley, rice, chives, celery, lettuce and sunflower seeds

Dill, borage flowers and chives are herbs traditionally used to improve fingernails. They can be used externally as a finger bath.

Make a strong infusion of one of the 'fingernail herbs' in a ceramic bowl, steep overnight, strain and store in the refrigerator for up to 5 days.

A suggested strength would be 9 tablespoons of fresh herb (or 3 teaspoons of dried herb) in 300 ml of boiling water.

Soak your fingertips in the solution for 15 minutes morning and night. To keep your fingernails supple, massage a little olive oil into them each night after using the herbal nail bath.

# Hangover

Drinking plenty of lemon juice in water (or orange juice, for extra vitamin C), or hot peppermint or thyme tea can alleviate the discomfort of hangover. A herbal tea of equal parts yarrow and elder flower will help eliminate toxins from your body.

*See also Overindulgence, Thyme.*

# Hawthorn

Hawthorn (*Crataegus oxyacantha*) has been shown to be a cardiac tonic in organic and functional heart problems, and is reputed to help relieve hypertension, cardiac arrhythmias, arteriosclerosis, angina pectoris, palpitations, and diseases of the heart valves. Both the flowers and berries are astringent and useful in a decoction to ease sore throats.

Hawthorn capsules and tablets are available from health food stores.

# Hay Fever

Hay fever is triggered by things such as house dust, foods, feathers, industrial fumes and polluted air.

Herbal solutions have been used for centuries to provide relief from hay fever. Garlic and echinacea provide antimicrobial support to keep the many bugs that flourish in our mucus-filled sinuses under control. Horseradish helps remove mucus from the nasal and sinus passages, while fenugreek helps soothe irritated nasal and sinus tissues, and also helps to dry up the catarrh that allergy sufferers are prone to.

Herbs for hay fever relief are available in supplement form from health food stores. For watery and itchy eyes, congested sinuses and a runny nose, look for a sinus and catarrh complex containing horseradish and garlic.

Your diet should also include plenty of fresh fruit and vegetables, such as apples, figs, lemons, oranges, mandarins, peaches, carrots, raw grated beetroot, celery, cauliflower, onions, green peppers, turnips and young dandelion greens (lightly steamed or raw in a salad). Other beneficial foods are barley and raisins. Avoid all refined foods, especially wheat flour products, alcohol and carbonated drinks. Milk products should be used sparingly and with caution; replace them with soya substitutes.

## INHALANT REMEDY

Add 3 drops of rosemary oil and 1 drop each of thyme and peppermint oil to a bowl of boiling water. Lean over the bowl, cover your head with a large towel so as to form a tent and inhale the vapour for approximately 10 minutes each evening. People prone to high blood pressure, heart problems, asthma or other breathing difficulties, and those with sensitive or broken skin, should avoid this treatment unless advised otherwise by a health practitioner.

For a convenient inhalant that can be used anywhere, blend together 2 drops of rosemary oil and 1 drop each of geranium and eucalyptus oil. Put 1 drop of the oil blend on a tissue or handkerchief and inhale whenever needed to ease laboured breathing and a stuffy nose.

*See also Allergies, Nasal Congestion, Sinusitis.*

# Headache

The causes of headaches are numerous, but whatever the cause, they are usually associated with a great deal of discomfort. There are a number of simple remedies you may wish to try next time a headache persists; however, an increase in the intake of calcium may help prevent them.

## MINOR HEADACHES

Put a couple of drops of lavender oil on your fingertips and massage into your temples and the base of your skull. Lavender oil rubbed into the wrists and the nape of the neck also has a calming effect.

## NAGGING HEADACHES

To ease a nagging headache, try a cup of meadowsweet tea. Aspirin is found in this plant. Make your meadowsweet tea using 1 tablespoon of fresh herb or 1 level teaspoon of dried herb to 300 ml of boiling water. Drink one cupful as needed, but no more than 3 cups a day.

## GASTRIC HEADACHES

These are usually caused by eating the wrong foods. Mix 1 drop of peppermint oil with a teaspoon of honey and dissolve in 1 cup of warm water. Sip slowly while you sit back and relax.

## MIGRAINE HEADACHES

The herb feverfew (*Tanacetum parthenium*) is an extremely good preventive for migraine headaches. Eat 3 leaves of the fresh herb every day, in a sandwich or wrapped in a piece of bread (it is best not to chew the fresh leaf), or take feverfew capsules (available from health food stores), or drink a cup of feverfew tea. Be careful, though: feverfew can cause mouth dryness and mouth ulcers, irritation and pain in highly sensitive people.

Take $\frac{1}{2}$ cup of feverfew tea every hour at the first sign of migraine attack or tension, or 1 cup every morning as a preventive. You can buy feverfew tea from health food stores or, if you prefer, you can make it fresh from the herb. To make fresh feverfew tea use 1 tablespoon of the fresh herb to 300 ml of boiling water. For individual cups, pour in the hot water, cover, infuse for 3 minutes, and strain into another cup. If brewing in a teapot, allow 1 serve per individual and 1 for the pot. Infuse for 5 minutes in boiling water, then strain into individual cups. Brew the tea only in a ceramic teapot.

## TENSION HEADACHES

Put a few drops of lavender oil in a bowl of warm water, wring out a handkerchief in it and apply to the back of the neck.

Rosemary oil is also excellent for treating this type of headache, especially one that is throbbing in the temples and causes squinting of the eyes. Massage a few drops of the oil on your temples and across your forehead, and then gently down and around your jawbone. The nerves of your face will quickly relax and the headache will ease.

A warm footbath and massage to the upper back, shoulders and neck will often help.

## PRE-MENSTRUAL HEADACHE

To help pre-menstrual headaches, take evening primrose oil. The capsules are available from health food stores and should be taken as directed on the label.

---

*See also Chamomile, Floral Vinegar, Herbal Teas, Lavender, Menstrual Problems.*

# Head Lice

Head lice and nits can become a real problem in schools and other places where there are groups of children. Herbs and essential oils can control lice, and are far more gentle to humans than many of the chemical concoctions normally used.

These tiny insects love living in human hair and are usually passed on from one person to another by direct contact. Sharing of brushes, hats, pillows, etc. will also spread them. Head lice aren't fussy about whose hair it is they're living in — all they want is a nice warm home to lay their eggs in.

Lice puncture the skin and suck blood, laying eggs, called nits, which attach to the hair. Itching of the head is the first sign that someone may have lice and nits, but itching doesn't start until these insects are in some numbers and have been in residence for a couple of months. Thoroughly check the hair, looking close to the scalp — the grey eggs are only just visible to the naked eye. However, they are clearly visible with a magnifying glass.

Combing essential oil of thyme through the hair with a fine-toothed comb daily, until the problem clears up, is a natural remedy. Thyme is a powerful antiseptic which contains thymol; it will help control nits (*see Thyme*).

An old-fashioned treatment that I found extremely effective when my son was 9 years old is a hair rinse made from quassia (pronounced kwarsha) chips. Some chemists may still stock quassia chips. If not, they can order them in for you; herbal suppliers and some health food or specialty shops may also be able to help.

To make the lice rinse, boil 15 g of quassia chips in 2 litres of water in an enamel or stainless steel pan for 2 hours, topping up the liquid if necessary. Strain and add 1 tablespoon of cider vinegar to every 300 ml of liquid. Apply by combing through the hair with a very fine-toothed comb. Repeat at 2-week intervals, 4 times altogether.

Another very effective treatment is to apply a blend of the following essential oils: 25 drops each of rosemary and lavender, 15 drops geranium and 12 drops eucalyptus, thoroughly mixed with 75 ml of almond oil.

Divide the hair into small sections and saturate each section with the mixture down to the roots. Pile long hair on top of the head, ensuring that every bit is oiled. Wrap plastic around the head and behind the ears to stop the oils evaporating. (With small children, be careful that they cannot move the plastic anywhere near their noses or mouths and thus restrict their breathing.) Leave for 2 hours, then remove the plastic and wash the hair, rubbing the shampoo in well. Rinse thoroughly and comb through with a fine-toothed comb. Repeat 3 days later.

*See also Thyme.*

# Health-Giving Juices

*See Juices for Health.*

# Heartburn

Drinking a cup of peppermint tea or chewing on a mint leaf will give speedy relief.

*See also Digestion, Indigestion.*

# Heat Exhaustion

This is caused by not drinking enough water in hot weather and losing salt from the body. Symptoms include feeling dizzy, faint or nauseous, and sometimes — but not always — thirsty.

Get out of the sun immediately and drink as much water as you can.

When travelling, or if you are likely to have to spend time outdoors in hot weather, drink at least 3 litres of water a day. Add 1 teaspoon of salt per litre to the water. Carry a bottle of lavender or eucalyptus oil with you in case of heatstroke. Apply this to your temples, the back of your neck and your solar plexus, and breathe deeply — this will help ease symptoms.

*See also Sun Protection, Sunstroke.*

# Herbal Detox

Overwork, long hours and stress play havoc with our bodies, and tend to slow down our thinking. When this happens, it's time to do a little gentle housekeeping by cleansing the body with herbs. Not only will you have renewed energy and mental clarity, but you will also feel that you can tackle life again. The regime will cleanse your system, boost your liver function and promote good digestion.

For best results, you should stick to the detoxification regime for 7 days. During this period eat plenty of fruit, vegetables and wholegrain foods. Avoid processed foods, red meat, alcohol and caffeine.

Each morning, before eating, drink a 250 ml glass of water with the juice of ½ lemon. (Lemon stimulates gastric juices and acts as a mild laxative.) Next, dissolve 1 tablespoon of psyllium husk powder (available from health food stores) in another glass of water and drink it. Finish your morning routine with a glass of plain water.

At breakfast, lunch and dinner take milk thistle (*Silybum marianum*) tablets or capsules (as directed on the label). These are also available from health food stores.

Four times a day, between meals, drink 1 cup of the following herbal tea:

*4 tablespoons dried dandelion root*
*1 tablespoon dried licorice root*
*1 tablespoon unpeeled fresh ginger*
*½ tablespoon fennel seeds*
*7 cups water*

Place the herbs and water in an enamel or stainless steel pan. Cover, bring to the boil, then simmer for 15 minutes. Remove from heat and allow to infuse and cool to room temperature. Strain into a ceramic cup and drink, refrigerating any leftovers. Reheat leftovers to room temperature before drinking.

You will need to make a fresh batch of this herbal tea each day.

*See also Fasting.*

# Herbal Teas

Since ancient times, herbal teas have been used to ease certain ailments. Today they are just as appropriate — they also provide a refreshing taste alternative to conventional teas.

Most of the herbs you need are available from health food stores, some chemists and even supermarkets. However, fresh is best! Why not start your own herbal tea garden?

Teas are made from the leaves, flowers, seeds, berries, bark or root of various herbs. A herbal tea is no more than an infusion of fresh or dried herbs with boiling water. In some cases a single part of the plant exerts the most beneficial effect; other teas require a combination of plant parts.

A herbal tea can be drunk at any time of the day, either hot or iced, and taken with the addition of honey, a slice of lemon, or a tablespoon of rosewater. Some herbal teas, taken over a long period of time, help build resistance to various illnesses and conditions. Their benefits are generally cumulative rather than instantaneous. However, remember that herbs are, in their own way, potent, and therefore must be used carefully.

To make your herbal tea, unless otherwise directed on the packet, brew as you would conventional tea, infusing herbal tea bags for 3 minutes or steeping the dried or fresh herbs in a teapot. Put 1 level teaspoon of dried herb, or 1 tablespoon of fresh herb, for each individual cup into a teapot, plus one for the pot, and pour in boiling water. Infuse for 5 minutes, then strain into cups. Use only ceramic, enamel or stainless steel teapots.

## ALFALFA

Alfalfa has a bland taste, but is quite acceptable when blended with mint, lemon verbena and/or honey. It is a rich source of iron, phosphorus, potassium and magnesium. It is thought to relieve arthritis and other twinges and pains, and to improve digestion.

## CINNAMON

For something a little different, why not try cinnamon tea! This delicious, spicy tea is a favourite with my family, especially on cold winter nights. Put 250 g of dried clover blossoms and 1 large cinnamon stick, broken into pieces, in an enamel or stainless steel pan and add half a litre of boiling water. Bring to a simmer, add 1 teaspoon of finely grated orange rind and cook gently for 5 minutes. Remove from heat, cover the pan, and infuse for a further 5 minutes. Strain and sweeten to taste with honey. Any excess cinnamon tea can be stored in the refrigerator for up to 3 days and warmed before drinking.

## CHAMOMILE

Chamomile is one of the safest and gentlest of all the herbs. It has a light, apple-like taste and is rich in calcium.

It is used to soothe gastro-intestinal disorders, relieve menstrual pain, reduce fever and restlessness in children, and is said to induce sound, natural sleep and to calm an overactive brain. In Europe many people drink a cup of this herbal tea as their customary 'nightcap', to relax them before going to bed. It will also expel worms, help teething children, and help in the treatment of children with red, inflamed eyes (when used as an eye bath or compress).

## FEVERFEW

*See Feverfew, Headaches (Migraine).*

## LEMON BALM

Drinking lemon balm tea during hot weather will help lessen the effects of exhaustion. It is very refreshing and makes an excellent cold drink when mixed with fresh fruit juice. This tea will help digestion and help stimulate the appetite, aid in settling an upset stomach and help ease griping stomach pains.

## LEMON GRASS

An excellent first herbal tea to try, if you have not already enjoyed the experience, is lemon grass. It is very palatable and refreshing, rich in vitamin A, and is considered ideal for purifying the skin and refining its texture.

## NETTLE

Nettle has a very bland taste, and should be drunk with a little mint or honey. The tea contains vitamin D, iron, calcium and other trace elements. It is traditionally used as a blood tonic, and to stimulate digestion and increase lactation in nursing mothers. It is said that its astringent qualities will relieve urinary disorders, rheumatic problems and colds.

## PEPPERMINT

Peppermint has a refreshing and delicately fruity taste, and is one of the best known of the herbal teas. It acts as a tonic and is reputed to relieve chest congestion and congestion in any part of the body. It relieves indigestion, flatulence and digestive disturbances, and acts as a mild sedative when taken before going to bed. Add a slice of lemon and honey and drink it to help ease a nagging headache. Blended with equal parts of yarrow and elder flower, it is a time-tested remedy for colds. Drink 1 cup every 2 hours to help relieve symptoms.

## ROSEHIP

Rosehip tea has always been a very popular beverage for prevention of colds. It is an excellent source of vitamin C, as well as of vitamins A, E and B. It can be drunk hot in winter with a slice of lemon, a little honey and a pinch of spice, or iced in summer with sprigs of spearmint or peppermint, honey, ice cubes and slices of lemon.

## ROSEMARY

Rosemary has a fragrant, aromatic taste. It has long been revered as an all-purpose tonic that freshens breath, induces sleep, alleviates headaches and strengthens the nerves. The cooled tea can be rubbed into the scalp as a hair tonic.

## SAGE

Sage leaf has a stimulating, slightly bitter taste. It has a long history of use for rheumatic complaints, calming the nerves, soothing a sore throat (gargle) and as a tonic for the liver and brain.

## SUBSTITUTE FOR CONVENTIONAL TEA

Natural herbal blends contain no caffeine or tannin, both of which are very strong stimulants. A blend of red clover flower, dandelion leaf and peppermint leaf is the perfect introduction for those people who are used to drinking ordinary tea.

Blend equal portions of the dried herbs and store until needed in an airtight glass container away from direct light and heat.

To make the tea, put 1 level teaspoon of dried herb for each individual cup into a ceramic teapot, plus one for the pot, and pour in boiling water. Infuse for 5 minutes, then strain into cups.

## TEAS FOR SPECIFIC COMPLAINTS

The following lists the teas that can be used for specific complaints — either on their own or as a mixture.

- Tonic — borage, sage, mint, rosemary, dandelion, blackberry, raspberry or strawberry leaf.
- Infections, coughs and colds — angelica, elder flower, yarrow, peppermint, thyme, rosehip, aniseed, horehound, fenugreek or lemon grass.
- Cooling the body and reducing fever — lemon balm, borage, peppermint, elder flower or yarrow.
- For the liver — angelica, parsley or fenugreek.

- For the kidneys and as a diuretic — celery seed, dandelion or parsley.
- Indigestion, stomach ache and flatulence — dill, peppermint, caraway, fennel, aniseed, lovage, rosemary, chamomile, coriander, sage, thyme, spearmint or lemon balm.
- Nausea — dandelion, spearmint, peppermint or basil.
- Rheumatic pain — parsley, angelica or celery.
- Mild sedative, relaxation — linden (lime) flower, chamomile or lemon verbena.

## Herbal Vinegar

*See Floral Vinegar.*

## Hiccups

Take 1 cup of aniseed tea or 1 teaspoon of powdered aniseed as needed. A little dill water (*see **Dill***) will also help relieve hiccups.

My grandmother recommended sucking a lump of sugar soaked in vinegar. However, you may prefer to add 2 or 3 drops of peppermint or cinnamon oil.

## High-Protein Mixed Salad

This high-protein mixed vegetable salad makes a perfect summer meal that is both delicious and nutritious; it is ideal for busy people on the go or those who work hard or play hard.

To make the salad you will need 1 cup each of fresh broccoli and fresh beans, 500 g of ricotta cheese, broken into small pieces, 2 tomatoes, cut into bite-sized pieces, 1 celery stalk, chopped, 1 small red capsicum, cut into fine strips, 3 lettuce leaves, torn into pieces, and 4 tablespoons of sunflower seed kernels.

Lightly steam the broccoli and beans, then place all the ingredients, except the sunflower seeds, in a salad bowl and toss. You will find that the ricotta cheese becomes the salad dressing. Sprinkle the sunflower seeds on top of the tossed salad, and serve.

*See also Energy Fruit Salad.*

# Honey

Honey was known to the ancient Greeks as the food of the gods because of its unique healing properties. It has always been used for rejuvenating purposes. It contains many vitamins and minerals — many of the B group vitamins, vitamin C, carotene and organic acids. It works well as a natural skin softener, an antiseptic, and is also an ideal ingredient for natural skin care preparations.

Honey cleanses, heals and moisturises the skin, easily removing dead cells. It is very effective for treating dry, chapped skin and windblown or damaged lips.

When using honey on the skin it is best to use natural unprocessed honey, not honey that has been boiled excessively during processing.

Here are a few ideas that will help you nurture yourself with honey and keep you feeling and looking good.

To clean facial skin, mix together equal amounts of clear honey and wheat germ oil and spread it over your face, avoiding your eyes. Keep it on for 15 minutes, relaxing while you wait. Wash it off with lukewarm water and then splash cold water on your face to close your pores. Pat your face dry with a soft towel. This mixture is also especially effective for removing blackheads.

For hands that have been excessively exposed to harsh climatic conditions use this rich, oily overnight conditioner. Gently warm together in a double boiler 1 teaspoon of honey and 1 tablespoon each of almond oil and olive oil. Stir constantly until well blended. Remove from heat and beat in 2 teaspoons of glycerine. Bottle and seal.

Massage the lotion well into your hands, then put on a pair of cotton gloves for increased absorption.

If you are one of the many people who suffer with dry flaky skin on their feet, daily use of a honey treatment will help alleviate this problem. First splash warm water on your feet, then rub in a good layer of honey and leave for about ½ hour so that it is well absorbed into your skin. Rinse residual honey off with warm water and pat dry. Continue this remedy daily until the condition of your feet improves.

Honey is also great for insomniacs. Just take a teaspoon at bedtime — the sugars in honey stimulate serotonin production, which induces relaxation. You'll soon nod off into a natural, restful sleep.

_See also Skin Care, Sleep._

# Honeysuckle

For centuries, poets have sung the praises of honeysuckle's beauty and sweet perfume, creating images of sun-filled, lazy summer days. Honeysuckle is an 'old-world' plant that should be included in every herb garden, climbing beautifully up a trellis or just rambling across the back fence.

Culpeper, the great seventeenth century herbalist, regarded honeysuckle as _'a hot martial plant in the sign of Cancer, the leaves being put into gargarisms for sore throats'_, and it was one of the plants Dioscorides, a famous Greek physician and plant expert of the first century AD, recommended for curing hiccups. Later, in the 1500s, celebrated English herbalist John Gerard listed the virtues of honeysuckle too: _'the floures steeped in oil and set in the Sun, are good to anoint the body that is benummed, and growne very cold'_. And it was one of those flowers listed by Francis Bacon in the seventeenth century in his essay _Of Gardens_: its _'breath'_ is _'far sweeter in the air than in the hand'_.

## HONEYSUCKLE SYRUP

This is a good syrup to use for the relief of sore throat. Sip 15 ml whenever required.

*2¹/₂ cups fresh honeysuckle flowers*
*1¹/₄ cups boiling water*
*¹/₂ cup sugar*

Lightly crush and bruise the honeysuckle petals before pouring the hot water over them. Set them aside to cool, then strain the liquid through muslin into an enamel or stainless steel saucepan, making sure to squeeze and keep all liquid from the petals. Add the sugar and bring slowly to the boil, then simmer gently until the mixture is of a syrupy consistency. Cool slightly, then pour into a sterilised bottle and seal.

## HONEYSUCKLE OINTMENT

This delightfully fragrant but gentle ointment can be used on minor burns and sunburn.

*3 heaped tablespoons fresh honeysuckle petals*
*¹/₂ cup petroleum jelly*

Crush and bruise the honeysuckle flowers. Put them, and the petroleum jelly, in a small ceramic bowl in a pan of boiling water. Simmer for 20 minutes, stirring occasionally, then strain into a warm sterilised glass jar and leave to cool. Seal and label.

# Horseradish

When included regularly in the diet, horseradish (*Armoracia rusticana*) is a remedy for sinus, repeated nasal colds and bronchial complaints. It will also provide relief for sufferers of rheumatism and gout, and acts a diuretic. Used externally as an ointment it makes an excellent rub to disperse congestion from a cold.

Horseradish is available in tablet form from health food stores or as a whole root from a greengrocer.

*See also Colds, Herbal Chest Rub.*

# Hygiene

If we shower daily and wear clean clothes, applying expensive toiletries designed to mask body odours is usually unnecessary. However, sometimes Nature does need a little help, and something as simple and inexpensive as a herbal deodorant, which will control unpleasant odour without inhibiting perspiration, is all that is needed.

A light dusting of bicarbonate of soda under the arms is simple, safe and effective. Or a solution of bicarbonate of soda and water can be poured into a refillable roll-on bottle and used like a purchased roll-on deodorant.

An effective herbal deodorant can be made with herbs and cider vinegar. It will have both a subdued perfume and antiseptic properties, and will keep you feeling fresh and odour free. Herbs suitable to use in a liquid deodorant are rosemary, thyme, lavender, sage, lovage, eau-de-cologne mint, spearmint, scented geranium (Pelargonium) leaves, eucalyptus, marjoram and honeysuckle flowers. The scented geraniums, which are easy to propagate and grow in most climates, provide a varying range of fragrances and are ideal as deodorant herbs.

Other common natural deodorant fragrances include nutmeg, rose, coconut, lime, apple-scented mint and peppermint.

## NATURAL DEODORANT

To make your herbal deodorant, place 3 tablespoons of dried herb or 6 tablespoons of dried flower petals in a ceramic bowl. If it's more convenient to use fresh herbs and flowers, double the quantity. Mix together 300 ml each of apple cider vinegar and distilled water and, in an enamel or stainless steel saucepan, heat to just below boiling point. Pour the liquid over the herbs, cover tightly with plastic wrap and leave to steep for 12 hours. Strain and dilute 50/50 with distilled water if you find the fragrance too strong. Store in a bottle with a tight-fitting lid. After washing and drying under your arms, dab on the natural deodorant and allow it to dry.

# I

## Indigestion

Many of the herbs best known and most used for flavouring and seasoning stimulate the flow of digestive juices in the stomach and intestines. Classic herb and food partnerships in cooking reflect this: rosemary helps the digestion of fatty lamb; fennel assists the digestion of oily fish; horseradish aids in the digestion of beef.

Aromatic seeds such as aniseed, cardamom, caraway, dill and fennel are useful digestives. A tablespoon of ground aniseed boiled in a cup of milk and drunk twice a day will improve digestion. To increase the flow of saliva, add 1 teaspoon of cardamom to the aniseed drink and take 1/2 hour before meals.

However, it is important to remember not to eat while your stomach is upset. You can eat light foods once treatment has commenced, but only when you feel some form of appetite. Don't eat for the sake of eating. Acceptable types of food are porridge, light vegetable soup, salads, a small amount of toasted wholemeal bread, grated apple and rice.

If you suffer from indigestion, a simple remedy to help ease it is to dissolve 1/2 teaspoon of bicarbonate of soda in a glass of hot water, and sip it slowly. Or take 2 drops of nutmeg oil blended with 1 teaspoon of honey after each meal as a preventive. Another treatment is to add 1 drop of peppermint essential oil to a glass of warm water, with a little honey, and sip slowly. This acts extremely quickly. It will also counteract nausea during pregnancy.

Peppermint and rosemary tea is also helpful in easing indigestion. Steep 1 teaspoon of each of the dried herbs in 1 cup of boiling water for approximately 3 minutes, and then strain the liquid into another cup. Reheat if required, add a slice of lemon and sweeten with honey. Drink 1 cup morning and night. One cup of peppermint tea first thing every morning is another good preventive remedy.

Vegetables that will help relieve this problem are raw cabbage and raw potato. Simply liquidise ½ cabbage and 1 potato, and then press the liquid through a fine wire sieve. Dilute 1 cup of the juice with ½ cup of cooled boiled water and sip slowly throughout the day.

To help prevent indigestion include herbs and spices such as coriander, fennel and aniseed in your cooking. A glass of fresh carrot juice each morning on rising will also help regulate your digestive process. And to prevent embarrassing wind, include oranges in your daily diet.

Persistent indigestion should be investigated by your health practitioner.

---

*See also Acidity, Dill Water, Herbal Teas, Medicinal Food,*
  *Overindulgence, Stomach, Thyme.*

# Insect Bite Itch

Apply neat apple cider vinegar to the itchy spot, or add 500 ml of apple cider vinegar to a warm bath and soak in it. Lavender oil and tea-tree oil are also effective remedies, so keep a bottle of either in the car or handbag on family outings.

---

*See also Itchiness, Stings and Bites.*

# Insomnia

All of us at some time have one of those nights where we toss and turn and just can't sleep. Fatigue, tension, anxiety, overexcitement and pain are some of the causes of sleepless nights.

▶ If you have had a hectic day, relax at night and avoid evening activities that are mentally demanding.

▶ Don't bring your work home from the office.

- Drink a cup of chamomile tea instead of coffee after dinner, and another cup ½ hour before going to bed.
- If you're really wound up, relax in a soothing and calming warm herbal bath. Herbs you can use in the bath are bay leaf, chamomile, hyssop, lemon balm, lime (linden) flowers, lovage, pennyroyal, rosemary, valerian and yarrow. Put 2 tablespoons of dried herbs of your choice in the centre of a 20 cm square of muslin. Draw up the sides and secure them with a piece of ribbon, then hang them under the running tap so that the water gushes through it (*see Bathing*).

However, if you continually suffer from insomnia, your diet may be inadequate and you may not be getting sufficient vitamins and minerals to soothe your nerves and tone up your nervous system. If your calcium and magnesium intake is insufficient, take a daily supplement, available from health food stores. Your diet should include apples, almonds, barley, cabbage, celery, leeks, lettuce, fresh sliced mushrooms, onions, peas, baked potatoes, brown rice, soya beans, spinach, sweet corn, turnips and tomatoes.

A cup of valerian tea an hour before going to bed can help you re-establish a normal sleep cycle, and is safe to take in conjunction with any prescribed medication. However, valerian has an off-putting taste, so blend it with equal amounts of a better-tasting herb such as mint. You can also add honey to taste, if required.

A drop of lavender oil on your pillow will help promote sound, natural sleep. You can also try basil, chamomile, juniper, neroli or sandalwood essential oil.

## SLEEP PILLOWS

Pillows stuffed with sweet-scented grasses or herbs have been used over the centuries to induce natural, restful sleep.

The simplest and easiest way to provide yourself with a sleep pillow is to make a herb bag, of whatever size you require, to slip inside your pillowcase. The herb bag can be made from either muslin, cheesecloth, cotton or linen, and then filled with the appropriate sleep herbs.

Dried hops, with its soft, sweet smell, is an excellent choice. Sweet-scented woodruff and southernwood mixed with hops will quickly lull you into a restful sleep. For a sharper scent, add rosemary and bay leaf; for a more soothing, clean scent, try peppermint and lemon balm.

Lavender is very refreshing, and especially delightful when mixed with rose petals. Never mix it with hops, however, as the two do not go together.

Marjoram, when mixed with woodruff, agrimony and southernwood, will give you a delicate, sweet scent and a restful sleep. Other herbs to use for their sleep-inducing properties are: angelica, bergamot, clover, chamomile, dill, lime flowers, lemon balm, rosemary, sage and thyme.

Spices can also be included in sleep pillow mixes. Cloves will help clear your head, and are reputed to prevent snoring. Other spices which will give the mix a sweet or tangy perfume are cinnamon, allspice, lemon and orange peel, orrisroot and pine needles.

---

*See also Chamomile, Lavender, Sleep.*

# Iodine

Iodine is a vital element in the health and correct activity of the thyroid gland. This gland directly or indirectly controls every metabolic process, so good function must be maintained to keep the endocrine system in a state of balance and health.

Kelp is the greatest natural source of iodine.

# Iron

Iron is vital to the growth of any living organism. It not only burns up a lot of garbage, it regenerates as well, transporting oxygen to every cell in the body.

Women are more likely to be deficient in iron than men. In each menstrual period they use 15–30 mg of iron. If this loss is not overcome by including high natural sources of iron in the diet, anaemia can result.

In the animal protein group, red meat is the richest source of this mineral, followed by chicken and fish. However, iron can also be obtained from other sources, an important factor to consider for vegetarians and those with high cholesterol problems. There is an abundance of it found in all the green leafy vegetables, particularly in the darker leaves. Iron is also in high concentration in some seeds, particularly in the germ of wheat. A generous spoonful of wheat germ sprinkled over your breakfast cereal will almost be enough for your daily requirement.

Natural unprocessed bran gives you plenty of iron and tones up your bowels as well. Pumpkin seeds, dried and fresh, are high in this mineral, and sesame seeds follow not far behind. Herbal teas, such as alfalfa and yellow dock, will add to your iron intake and soya beans are exceedingly rich in it, as are most of the bean family.

Oatmeal is good iron food and will give you a good start to the day. You can get your daily ration from your porridge, if that's what you prefer. Add fresh seasonal fruit and some wheat germ and you have a super get-up-and-go breakfast. Egg yolks are acceptable, providing iron of animal origin that is easily assimilated.

Yogurt also contains this mineral. It is partly processed towards digestion and is therefore an excellent food to include in your diet if your digestion is weak, or if you are recovering from illness.

All leafy green vegetables, with the exception of spinach, which contains oxalic acid that inhibits the body from using the iron it contains, are a good source of this mineral.

Dandelion leaf, a common wild herb found growing almost everywhere, is rich in iron and also includes every other vital mineral needed by the body. Young leaves can be included in summer salads along with other greens, or cooked in the same way as spinach.

Iron is the mighty mineral that gives us the get-up-and-go to enjoy life.

*See also Eating for Health and Energy.*

# Irritability

*See Fatigue.*

# Itchiness

A peppermint bath is very soothing for itches. Put 4 teaspoons of dried peppermint in a ceramic bowl, add 500 ml of boiling water, cover and steep until cool. Strain through muslin cloth and add to bathwater.

A soda bath is marvellous for itching skin, for relief from vaginitis and for children who are allergic to bubble baths. Add ½ cup of bicarbonate of soda to your bath, swish it around until it dissolves, then lie back and relax.

An ointment made from chickweed and olive oil is excellent for treating itchy rashes. Simply simmer 1 cup of chickweed in ½ cup of olive oil for 20 minutes. Cool, strain and apply to the affected area as required.

Keep surplus ointment in a sterilised glass jar with a tight-fitting lid.

*See also Aloe Vera, Bathing, Eczema, Insect Bite Itch, Nettle Rash, Prickly Heat, Skin Irritations, Tea-Tree Oil.*

# J

## Jellyfish Sting

*See Insect Bite Itch, Stings and Bites.*

## Jet Lag

While flying, drink plenty of plain, still water and avoid alcohol, coffee and carbonated soft drinks. Most importantly, plan ahead. A week before take-off time, take a daily dose of Siberian ginseng capsules, as directed on the label; continue this same dosage for a week following arrival. If you have trouble relaxing or sleeping when you reach your destination, settle down with a cup of chamomile tea. Peppermint also helps allay nausea and acts as a soothing sedative to induce relaxation and sleep. Other mild sedative herbs are linden (lime flower) and lemon verbena.

*See also Travel Sickness.*

## Jiggers

*See Insect Bite Itch, Stings and Bites.*

## Jojoba

Jojoba (pronounced ho-ho-ba) is a traditional healing plant. The golden oil, or wax, extracted from its seed pod has many uses as a cosmetic oil, and its excellent lubricating qualities make it a fine moisturiser for the skin. Included in homemade moisturising creams it will moisturise and soften the skin, leaving it with a smooth, silky texture.

It can be used to treat such conditions as dry scalp, psoriasis and eczema. Jojoba also conditions your hair; it is an ingredient in many familiar store-bought soaps and shampoos.

Practical uses for jojoba oil at home are:

- Pure cold-pressed jojoba oil can be applied to all types of skin. Apply a few drops directly onto chapped or sore lips, dry skin or general skin disorders such as eczema, psoriasis, dandruff or acne. If applied lightly, it can act as a fine facial moisturiser.
- It is a valuable adjunct to your usual skin protection regime in summer; it does not actually prevent sunburn, but it helps your skin retain moisture, and can be used in conjunction with sun-blocking creams.
- Use it to treat persistent warts — add a drop of oil to the affected spot morning and evening.
- Eat a few ground or roasted jojoba beans each morning to strengthen a weak stomach and relieve acidity, but don't take excessive amounts. Large quantities can have a purgative effect.
- Because jojoba contains anti-inflammatory myristic acid, it also has the potential to relieve rheumatism and arthritis. Rub the oil directly into sore joints whenever required.

# Joints, Painful

Cabbage leaves will ease hot, painful joints. Slightly bruise the leaves, apply to the affected joint, bind in position and leave on overnight.

A vinegar compress is also effective. Dip a clean cloth into hot apple cider vinegar, wring out slightly to stop it dripping, and apply as hot as you can tolerate.

*See also Aching Joints and Muscles, Bathing, Chamomile, Muscular Aches and Pains.*

# Juices for Health

Juices are a great way to top up your vitamin and mineral supply. They can be used pure or blended for a health-giving drink.

If you are using a blender to prepare your fruit and vegetable juices, peel and core fruit and strain after blending. If you are using a juice extractor, the fruit or vegetables can be left whole.

## PROPERTIES OF JUICES

| | |
|---|---|
| Apple | *Digestive; heals intestinal inflammation.* |
| Beetroot | *Blood builder.* |
| Cucumber | *Alkaliniser and mineraliser.* |
| Cabbage | *Source of vitamin U; natural source of healing for ulcers.* |
| Carrot | *Of all the juices, this is the best balanced in minerals and vitamins.* |
| Celery | *Natural nerve tonic.* |
| Dandelion | *Natural tonic for body fortification; blood builder; diuretic and source of organic magnesium for the teeth.* |
| Endive | *Rich in vitamins and minerals.* |
| Kale | *Rich in calcium and vitamins A, B and C.* |
| Parsley | *High in organic iron content; aids blood coagulation, eyes, glands and nerves.* |
| Orange | *Rich in calcium, vitamins A and C, and phosphorus.* |
| Tomato | *Rich in minerals.* |

The juice of wild and cultivated herbs also provides many healthy and delicious treats. If you find their juice too strong, blend it with carrot juice.

# JUICE DELIGHTS

### Apple and Cucumber Cooler

A cool and refreshing juice that is ideal for hot summer days.

2 apples
1/2 cucumber

Juice apples and cucumber in a juice extractor or blender and pour over ice cubes.

### Vitamin C Booster

2 oranges, peeled
2 pears
1 lemon

Process in a blender or juice extractor.

### Strawberry Delight

500 g watermelon, skin and seeds removed
155 g strawberries, hulled

Process in a blender or juice extractor.

### Vegetable Cocktail

A healthy pick-me-up first thing in the morning or after a busy day.

2 tomatoes
1 carrot
2 stalks celery
1 sprig fresh parsley

Process in a blender or juice extractor.

### Green Herbal Drink

See Bad Breath (Green Herbal Drink).

# K

## Kelp

Kelp is a mineral-rich health supplement that has many restorative properties. It is beneficial to your diet and to your overall health and sense of wellbeing. Kelp acts as a gentle tonic for the metabolism and a thyroid restorative, and is especially good for the adrenal and pituitary glands. It is rich in iodine, iron, trace minerals and nutrients, and when powdered kelp is mixed with fruit juice it makes a potent health drink that benefits the skin. Repeated small doses will decrease breast milk in nursing mothers. Quite often, herbalists will prescribe kelp for low thyroid activity and other symptoms of a sluggish constitution.

Kelp tablets and powder are available from health food stores.

**Warning:** *If kelp is not needed by the body, headaches may result from taking it. Take in combination with other herbs.*

## Kidneys

Always consult a medical practitioner for serious kidney malfunction and disorders.

Include the following in your diet as a preventive measure: fresh asparagus, avocado, cabbage, celery, freshly grated raw beetroot, fresh young dandelion greens, grapes, mangoes and pawpaw, radishes, squash (all types), strawberries and watermelon.

Drinking herbal teas is also beneficial, as well as drinking the water asparagus is cooked in. Beneficial herbal teas are: dandelion, parsley, celery, borage, nettle and alfalfa. Add a pinch of cayenne to the tea to speed up its beneficial effect and drink 1–6 cups a day. Dandelion tea is the ideal balanced diuretic, as it supplies potassium, a substance lost during diuretic action.

## Kiwi Fruit

The Chinese gooseberry (*Actinida chinensis*), commonly known as kiwi fruit, is a useful natural remedy. It is a good source of vitamin A, iron, some potassium and phosphorus, and has a higher vitamin C content than most citrus fruits.

It makes an ideal first food for babies and sick children, and for people recuperating from illness.

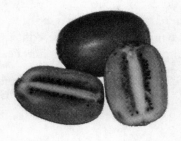

# L

## Laryngitis

Gargle as needed with sage tea. Other herbs that can be used as a throat gargle are garlic, thyme and fennel. Chilli is also an excellent gargle for laryngitis and sore throats, especially when combined with thyme and lavender.

### SAGE TEA

Infuse 15 g of dried tea leaves in 1 cup of boiling water (use a ceramic cup) for 10 minutes, then strain into another cup. Leave to cool and add honey to taste.

### LOSS OF VOICE

Drink 1 teaspoon of freshly squeezed parsley juice to $\frac{1}{2}$ cup of warm milk first thing in the morning.

*See also Chilli, Sage, Sore Throat.*

## Lavender

### THE FORGOTTEN HEALTH HERB

*The distiled water of Lavender cleaneth the sight and putteth away all spottes, lentils, freckles and redness of the face if they be often washed therewith.*

GERARD, HERBAL, 1597.

One of the best known and most loved of all the herbs, the many different varieties of lavender are grown in gardens everywhere, even when no special thought has been given to herbs as such. Lavender's use can be traced back to the Greeks and Romans, and today this highly aromatic herb has a myriad of health uses.

Added to bathwater lavender will relieve sore muscles and prevent skin dryness. Put 2 generous handfuls of dried lavender buds in a ceramic bowl. Mix together 500 ml each of distilled water and cider vinegar in a non-metallic saucepan and bring to just below boiling point. Pour the liquid over the herbs, seal the bowl with plastic wrap and allow to steep for 12 hours. Strain the mixture through fine muslin, squeezing and keeping all liquid from the herbs. Bottle for future use. Add 1 cup of lavender water to your bath while the water is running from the taps.

When colds and flu are around, lavender honey is a soothing and delicious herbal treat. Add a spoonful of the honey to a hot lemon drink and let its antiseptic qualities ease your sore throat.

Gently warm a bottle of light honey in a double boiler, add 1–2 tablespoons of dried lavender flowers (English lavender is best), and allow them to infuse for 2 minutes. Remove from the heat and allow to stand in the hot sun for a few hours — a sunny windowsill away from ants and other creatures is ideal. Strain out the lavender flowers and bottle.

Lavender tea is an ideal remedy for people with a gentle nature who suffer from headaches, migraine, dizziness and fainting spells. To prepare the tea, add 1 level teaspoon of dried flower heads to a ceramic cup, pour in hot water, cover, infuse for 3 minutes, and strain into another cup. Reheat if necessary.

If brewing in a teapot, allow 1 teaspoon per person and one for the pot. Pour on boiling water, infuse for 5 minutes then strain into individual cups. Use only a ceramic teapot, and set it aside for brewing only herbal teas.

If you suffer from insomnia, a drop of lavender oil on a pillowcase will exert a soporific effect and lull you to sleep.

Rubbed into the wrists or onto the nape of the neck, lavender oil has a calming effect.

Lavender essential oil can also be used in aromatherapy to ease headaches and to relax and calm the body.

*See also Colds, Headache, Herbal Teas, Insomnia, Medicinal Oils, Muscular Aches and Pains, Skin Care, Sleep.*

# Lemon Balm

The medicinal properties of lemon balm (*Melissa officinalis*) are numerous: it is a remedy for stomach upsets and eases griping pains, lessens the effects of exhaustion in hot weather and allays fainting spells, assists the digestion and improves the appetite, relieves sick feelings and acts as an anti-depressant. Lemon balm tea can also be used for scanty menstruation, as a nerve tonic, to ease palpitations of the heart, and for migraine headaches of a nervous origin. Spirit of balm can be applied to areas of bruising and painful rheumatic spots.

Lemon balm can be bought from most nurseries and is easy to grow in the home garden. It readily self-seeds each year, or large plant clumps can be divided at any time during the year.

### Spirit of Balm

*1 part (packed tight to equal 1 cupful of liquid in proportion) lemon balm leaves*
*3 parts vodka*
*3 parts water*

Put all ingredients in a glass jar, seal with an airtight lid and leave in a warm place for 2 days. Strain and store in an airtight bottle. Take 1 tablespoon in a glass of water, or as directed.

# Lice

*See Head Lice.*

# Licorice

This ancient herb has antiviral, antibacterial and anti-inflammatory properties, and is a well-known remedy for coughs and chest complaints generally, especially bronchitis. It is an ingredient in many popular cough medicines because of its soothing properties. It can also be taken as a tonic for lethargy, poor appetite, dry skin and hair. Dried licorice root is available at health food stores.

To make a tonic, infuse 30 g of the dried, chopped root in 300 ml of boiling water. Place the herb in a ceramic bowl, add the water, cover, and leave to infuse until it reaches room temperature. Strain and drink 1–3 cups of the tonic a day.

**Warning:** *Preparations containing licorice should be avoided during pregnancy and by people who have high blood pressure.*

# Liver

Serious and long-standing liver complaints should be treated by a health practitioner. However, both diet and herbs will help stimulate the liver and ease congestion.

Your diet should include apples, freshly grated raw beetroot, asparagus, cabbage, cauliflower, broccoli, spring onions, cucumbers, dates, lettuce, sweet corn, lemons, potatoes, raisins, sesame seeds, tomatoes, turnips, spinach, peaches and strawberries.

Of the herbs, dandelion is one of the most effective in treating liver complaints. It can be taken as a tea in all situations with complete safety. Drink 1 cup of tea 3 times a day. Other excellent herb teas are borage, celery, nettle, parsley, peppermint and rosemary. They will provide comfort and rapid relief from the results of overindulgence in alcohol or rich foods, and will also cleanse and stimulate a sluggish liver.

# Living Foods

Sprouts are a living food that will grow in any climate, and that rival meat in nutritional value. They can be cultivated at any time of the year, mature in 3–5 days, and require no soil or sunlight. They can be eaten raw, and have no waste.

Any live seed will sprout, though you must be careful to use only those that don't produce poisonous greens. Members of the 'nightshade family', such as tomatoes and potatoes, must be avoided. Vegetable seeds can also be sprouted for high nutrition food and will add variety to your diet. It is worth experimenting with any vegetable seed you happen to come across.

When buying seed for sprouting, insist on organically grown varieties, as they have the highest nutritional value. Or at least make sure that they haven't been treated with chemicals and are intended for sprouting. If you have a small patch of ground to spare, grow your own seed for sprouting. Your local agriculture department should be able to provide information on the planting and cultivation of various seed crops. Purchase good-quality seed with a minimum germination rate of 90 per cent, and buy in bulk — it's much cheaper.

When sprouting, avoid using containers made from soluble toxic metals such as copper, iron and aluminium. Almost anything else is acceptable, but I prefer to use various-sized glass containers.

All seed must be thoroughly washed and rinsed in fresh water. As a general guide, most seed is then soaked overnight in tepid water (at least 2 parts water to 1 part seed), but smaller seeds require a shorter soaking period; larger seeds need a longer soaking time. After the initial soaking, drain off the water and rinse the seed in fresh water.

The easiest and simplest way to sprout your seeds is to use a large preserving jar or coffee jar. Pierce a dozen or more holes in the lid, or stretch a piece of muslin cloth over the opening of the jar and hold it in place with a rubber band. A good rule of thumb for the amount of dried seed to be used is 1 tablespoon to a 1-litre jar.

Place the jar in a dark cupboard; sprouts grow more quickly as they search for sunlight. Immerse the jar in water and drain it 2–3 times a day until the sprouts are ready. With smaller seed you will need a fine mesh over the end of the jar, so as not to lose your seed.

Remove seed hulls daily, as they can cause sprouts to spoil.

If you wish to include chlorophyll in your sprouts, place them in a sunny spot after the first 3 days. Seeds that do well when grown for chlorophyll are fenugreek, alfalfa, radish and clover.

## SOYA BEANS

Soya beans require a slightly different preparation to get them to sprout.

First soak them overnight in warm water. Rinse, and remove any damaged seeds. Soak again overnight, then pour off the water and rinse. Keep in a dark cupboard and rinse 4–5 times a day. Be sure that no rinse water is left in the jar.

## SUPER ENERGY SPROUT BREAKFAST

This will provide nutrition and much needed energy throughout the day. Soak and sprout 2 handfuls of wheat seed. To avoid the sprout taste, eat the seed once the shoots are 2–3 mm in length, no longer.

Soak 1 handful each of sultanas and raisins overnight and reserve the soakwater. In the morning, combine 1 piece of finely chopped apple, 1 piece of finely diced seasonal fruit, 1 handful of ground mixed nuts, the sultanas and raisins, including the soakwater, your sprouts, and 1 tablespoon of fresh yogurt. Sprinkle with a pinch of powdered cinnamon and powdered vanilla bean.

# M

## Magnesium

Essential for the good health of the central nervous system, and indeed the whole of your body — magnesium is a mineral that makes you walk around feeling fully alive. It also plays an important role in hardening teeth and preventing tooth decay.

Natural sources of magnesium are alfalfa, almonds, apricots (dried), bananas, Brazil nuts, cashews and most other nuts, cabbage, celery, dandelion greens, dates (dried), fish, garlic, kelp, leafy green vegetables, molasses, parsley, potatoes cooked in their skins, prawns, radishes, sesame seeds, soya beans, sunflower seeds, tomatoes, watercress, wheat bran and wheat germ.

These foods should be included regularly in your diet as a preventive, to maintain your nervous system and keep it in tiptop condition.

## Margarine

See Butter and Margarine, Dietary Substitutes.

## Massage

Massage is important in many of the body's healing processes, and is invaluable for enhancing human health and vitality. The combination of touch and fragrance — the use of essential oils — can relieve stress and tension, alleviate fatigue and promote deep relaxation, as well as encourage the body's organs and systems to function at optimum levels. In a world filled with anxiety, massage is one obvious method of bringing comfort and consolation. It can quickly transport you from the rigours and problems of work and daily life, allowing you to feel renewed and refreshed.

Most of us feel tired and exhausted after a hectic day, but it is often not possible to have a full body massage. You can still revive your body and feel marvellous, though, with a foot, hand, self-body and facial massage.

## FEET

Before commencing a foot massage, blend 6 drops of either calendula or rosemary essential oil with 20 ml of almond oil.

*See also Feet.*

## HANDS

The pressure points of your hands can be worked for $\frac{1}{2}$ minute at a time. They are on the pads of each finger and the thumb, in the centre of the palm (this is known as the solar plexus point), and also slightly up and to the left (or right) of this point, between the thumb and little finger.

To massage, cradle one hand and support it with the fingers of your other hand, then apply pressure by alternately bending and straightening your thumb. For headaches, stress and neck pain, massage the pad of each thumb, from the knuckle joint to the tip, concentrating on the area closest to your forefinger.

Counteract fatigue by stimulating your adrenal glands. Treat both hands by applying pressure to the point slightly to the left (or right) of the solar plexus point. And if you have trouble unwinding or cannot sleep because of tension or racing thoughts, work the solar plexus point of both hands. Work each hand for at least 1 minute.

### HEAD COLD

Congested sinuses, and the dull, aching headache associated with them, can be relieved by working the reflex points (or pads) at the end of each finger.

## SELF-BODY MASSAGE

Pour 1 teaspoon of oil into your palm, rub your hands together, then apply it to your breasts and buttocks with a circular motion. Using a small amount of additional oil, rub your solar plexus 6 times in an anti-clockwise direction, then stroke the residual oil upwards on your stomach with both hands.

Add 1 more teaspoon of oil to your palm, rub your hands together, and massage each arm with firm strokes from the wrist to the shoulder. Finish by deeply, yet gently, kneading up your arm with your fingers.

Using 1 more teaspoon of oil, work upwards over your legs with deep, firm strokes. Massage from each ankle to the top of your thighs, working with both hands.

## SELF-FACIAL MASSAGE

Before starting the massage, ensure that your face has been thoroughly cleansed of grease, grime, dirt and make-up.

Pour 2 teaspoons of almond oil mix into a shallow saucer. Then place your hands in front of your face so that your fingers rest on your forehead and your thumbs rest just below your cheeks. Press gently and draw your fingers and thumbs towards your ears and away from your head. This helps release tension from your forehead.

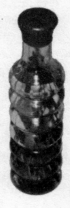

Dip your fingers lightly into the oil and gently rub your hands together. Using gentle strokes, start massaging under your chin, up over your face, and circle your eyes in an anti-clockwise direction (as you look at your fingers).

With a little more oil, gently massage your throat and up over your face again. Place your fingers at the centre of your forehead and begin light, yet firm, circular movements, massaging towards the temples and off at the hairline. Repeat this 2 or 3 times, finishing by pressing hard with your fingers on the middle of your forehead for a few seconds.

Massage behind your ears with small circular movements, and then press all around the outer ear, using the pads of the first two fingers.

Finish the massage by placing your thumbs on your chin and then, using gentle but firm pressure, pulling your thumbs along your jawbone to each ear. Do this 4 times.

*See also Eating for Health and Energy, Fatigue, Revitalisation, Spasmed Muscles, Stress and Tension.*

# Meat

Eating meat every day has become a normal part of a Western lifestyle, and meat has become our primary source of protein. However, the large consumption of meat is one of the major contributing factors to chronic and early degenerative disease.

It has long been argued that vegetarianism is the key to a healthier and happier life, and that the inclusion of meat in the diet is an invitation to a lifetime of diminished good health. This book has no intention of pursuing such an argument. The following advice is provided for those people who see animal meat as their principal protein source.

▶ Free-roaming animals, such as chickens or beef raised by non-commercial methods, will always be healthier than those commercially raised and chemically treated. Commercially raised chickens should be avoided, as they are often sick and carcinogenic.

▶ Consumption of animal meat should be reduced not only in quantity (per meal) but also in frequency. Because of the low vitamin content in meat, especially vitamins A and C, abundant salad vegetables, especially greens, should be included with the meal to facilitate maximum digestion.

▶ Fish caught within close proximity of industrial areas or farmland where there is a high use of chemical fertilisers, herbicides, etc. can also present health dangers.

# Medicinal Food

Did you know that a number of the fruits and vegetables we use almost daily in the kitchen have natural curative properties? This is no doubt why they have been used continually over the centuries as both food sources and natural medicines. They deserve a place among the other natural remedies and cures in this book, as they too contribute to the wellbeing of the body.

Without doubt, there is no better remedy than grated raw apple for general stomach upsets and gastric disturbances. It is especially good when taken after diarrhoea, as it will quickly restore the bowel function to normal.

When you're feeling tired and in need of a quick energy fix, try a banana. Mashed and mixed with a little honey and avocado, and served on oat biscuits, it makes a powerful energy-packed snack.

Lemons are well known for their antiseptic properties, and their juice makes an excellent gargle for a sore throat. As a fruity tingle, especially when included in cold and flu preparations, its mild sedative action will help reduce fever, as well as promoting the production of bile, which eases indigestion.

Oranges will stop embarrassing wind, as will eating 2 teaspoons of sugar-free, chunky marmalade with breakfast and main meals. Snacking on mandarins will calm irritated intestines, apples and pears will soothe your system when you are suffering from diarrhoea, and figs and prunes act as a mild laxative for constipation.

Watermelon is by far the most effective diuretic fruit, and is excellent for easing water retention and the bloated feeling that is often associated with the menstrual cycle.

Barley has long been known to have an anti-inflammatory action on the genito-urinary tract. To help reduce the discomfort of cystitis, try some old-fashioned barley water. To make your own barley water, simmer 50 g of unrefined barley (available from health food stores) in 1 litre of water for 40 minutes. Cool, strain, and drink over 24 hours. If the problem persists, consult your health practitioner.

Bran taken internally is an excellent remedy when you are recovering from an illness where there are signs of mineral deficiency, such as skin diseases. Add 2 tablespoons of bran to a pan and pour 2 cups (500 ml) of boiling water over it. Bring to the boil and simmer over a low heat for about 15 minutes, then strain. Take 1 cupful 3–5 times a day, as required.

Cabbage leaves can be used as a first aid measure to ease hot, painful joints, and cucumber soothes sore, inflamed skin. Raw beetroot juice can be taken for constipation, cystitis and skin diseases.

Carrot is rich in beta-carotene and numerous other beneficial substances. It will regulate the digestive process and help relieve constipation and diarrhoea. However, it must be taken in moderation, as an excess of beta-carotene will kill vitamin D in your body. One glass of the juice on rising is sufficient — in fact, limit your intake of carrot juice to 1 glass per day to enable your digestive juices to act upon the complex materials in the juice.

Celery is rich in vitamins A, B and C, and is helpful in easing laryngitis. Make a tea by steeping the leaves (not stalks) in boiling water for 10 minutes. Strain, cool, and mix half and half with milk. Drink a small glassful 3 times a day before meals; if you have laryngitis, gargle as required, then swallow.

Cucumber is rich in vitamin C, chlorophyll and mineral salts. It is reputed to cure migraines caused by menopause. Drink 1 small glass of cucumber juice a day.

French beans are beneficial to the heart, peas (which are rich in chlorophyll) sweeten the blood and improve circulation, and celery will exert a beneficial effect on the liver, kidneys, bladder, heart and nerves.

Common green garden peas, eaten daily in meals, will aid sufferers of varicose veins and haemorrhoids.

Garlic contains vitamins A, B and C, and copper, sulphur, manganese, iron and calcium. It is a natural antibiotic (if it is taken in large enough quantities), cleanses cholesterol and toxins from your bloodstream and stale mucus from your tissues, nourishes your nerves and increases glandular secretions.

Ginger is a natural antacid and aids in the elimination of colon gas. When added to bathwater it will open the pores of your skin and help rid your body of toxins.

Onion is an excellent disinfectant, a natural antibiotic, and is rich in vitamin B1. A regular intake ensures that your nervous system remains healthy.

Potato is reputed to be the most curative of all food remedies — this humble tuber contains vitamins A, B, D, E and H. A grated raw potato and 1 teaspoon of powdered ginger makes an excellent poultice for growths and skin infections, and a footbath of potato-peel water is a remedy for chilblains.

---

*See also Acidity, Eating for Health and Energy, Garlic, Indigestion, Overindulgence, Skin Irritations, Stomach.*

# Medicinal Oils

The medicinal properties of plant oils and their ability to deal with a wide range of first aid situations make them a useful addition to the home medicine cabinet. Because of their versatility it is not necessary to maintain a wide selection of them.

## CASTOR OIL

Castor oil is one of the best emergency remedies for drawing foreign bodies out of wounds. It will draw from up to 10 cm deep, thoroughly removing all the nasties. Use it as a poultice after stepping on a rusty nail, to draw out an abscess, a boil or any infection from any part of the body, and to draw out the infection of tick bites (including any part of the head that was left behind) and splinters.

The drawing action of castor oil is also very useful for removing splinters or other foreign bodies from the eye, allowing the offending bodies to be removed along natural channels.

## CHAMOMILE

Chamomile is very soothing, relaxing, calming and comforting to the nerves, and induces sound, natural sleep. It is the first choice for treating children's ailments: it can be used for teething troubles, in the bath to ease nerves and tetchiness, and in the treatment of red, inflamed eyes.

For general first aid it can be used in the treatment of burns (including sunburn), skin ailments such as psoriasis and eczema, sprains and strains, bruises, rashes, wounds, infections and windburn.

## EUCALYPTUS

Eucalyptus is highly aromatic, refreshing and head-clearing (it clears a stuffy nose to help you breathe more easily), and is an excellent oil for relieving muscular pain. It aids in the formation of skin tissue, and when massaged into your feet it will help induce deep sleep.

Its anti-inflammatory, antiseptic, antibiotic, deodorising and antiviral properties make eucalyptus oil a key addition to any basic kit of essential oils. In first aid situations, this oil is useful for animal bites, colds, grazes and cuts, infections, insect bites, itchy skin, overexercised muscles, sunburn and prickly heat, swellings and windburn.

## GERANIUM

This refreshing and relaxing oil is helpful for treating chilblains, blisters, muscle cramp, dry and flaky skin conditions, prickly heat and menstrual problems.

## LAVENDER

Lavender oil is a natural detoxifier, disinfectant, antiseptic and antibiotic which promotes healing and prevents scarring; it is especially effective for the treatment of burns and scalds.

Lavender oil is an excellent first aid remedy for insect bites and small burns, and its low toxicity makes it excellent for treating children's injuries. It can also be used to treat animal and insect bites, bruises, bumps, dry and flaky skin, blemished skin, grazes and cuts, infections, prickly heat, rashes, sprains and strains, swellings, wounds, muscular pain, headaches and windburn.

To treat a burn, first apply ice-cold water for at least 10 minutes. Then immediately put 2 drops of neat lavender oil directly onto the affected area. Put 5 drops of the neat oil on a dry, cold compress and cover the burn. Repeat as needed.

For blemished skin, first thoroughly cleanse your face, then mix 2 drops each of lavender oil and chamomile oil in the palm of your hands and massage it into your face. Leave on overnight.

If a blemish is coming up, dab on 1 drop of lavender oil to help it disappear.

## LINSEED

Linseed oil makes an ideal massage oil for treating sprained, strained, twisted, stretched and torn ligaments. It will ease tight muscles and ligaments and tone and improve elasticity in both tight and loose muscles.

Linseed oil is an essential sports medicine for the home first aid chest, to treat all those sprained ankles and twisted knees that seem to be an inherent part of growing up and playing sport.

## OLIVE OIL

Olive oil is useful for treating ears that tend to wax up or discharge, or ears that ache. If there is an infection deep in the ear, you can mix a bit of castor oil with the olive oil to add drawing power. Warm a little of the oil by putting a small jar of it in a pan of warm water. Add 3 drops to the affected ear and rub it in. Leave overnight, and clean with a bit of cotton wool the next morning. This treatment will not only clean the ears, it will also provide pain relief. For serious ear problems you should consult your family health practitioner.

Olive oil also acts as a soothing balm for all types of skin rashes, including those caused by an allergic reaction. A small amount of the warmed oil can be used to treat dry-scalp dandruff. Simply massage well into the scalp and leave for about 15 minutes, then wash out.

## PEPPERMINT

Peppermint has a refreshing scent that clears the head and improves breathing. It is a natural antiseptic and pain reliever, and can be used in the treatment of colds and flu, headaches, travel sickness, sunburn, toothache, indigestion and summer itch.

Because of its high potency, it must only be used in low concentrations (no more than 1 per cent) on inflamed or sensitive skin. High concentrations have a tendency to sting and burn the skin.

## ROSEMARY

Rosemary is an antiseptic oil that will relieve stiff joints and aching muscles, and is the perfect bath oil after a long, tiring day. Rosemary is excellent for maintaining healthy hair growth, controlling dandruff, aiding circulation, treating muscular sprains, arthritis and rheumatism, and helping to relieve fatigue and headaches (including migraine).

## TEA-TREE OIL

*See Tea-Tree Oil.*

## THYME

The powerful antiviral properties of this oil make it a vital component of any basic kit of essential oils. Its active ingredient is thymol — overuse can stimulate the thyroid gland and lymphatic system, so it should be used in moderation and is not suitable for children (unless otherwise directed by your health practitioner). Never apply thyme oil to the skin undiluted; blend it with an appropriate carrier oil first, such as almond oil or sunflower oil. Two or three drops to 5 ml of carrier oil should be sufficient.

This oil is especially useful for burning or including in an air freshener spray when colds and flu are around. It is also useful for treating respiratory problems, muscular pain, sprains and strains, and insect bites.

# Meditation

Anyone can meditate. It is a very simple way to forget about everyday stresses and concentrate solely on mental relaxation. During meditation the brain manufactures a balanced pattern of alpha and theta brainwave rhythms. This improved mental functionality leads to a healthier, more productive and fulfilled you. Practised regularly, meditation helps fight depression, hypertension, anxiety, migraine headaches and psychosomatic illnesses.

All you need is a quiet place where you know you'll be alone. If you spend all your waking hours preoccupied with work, you allow no time for yourself. We need to spend time alone with ourselves in silence, so that we can experience our aloneness and uniqueness, and rid our brains of accumulated clutter.

Begin today and experience the feeling of freedom that meditation will give you. You can start by simply sitting in a quiet place watching the wind in the trees, the clouds moving across the sky, or the sun setting — keep watching, without thinking, until you and the sky, the wind and the clouds become one.

If you live near the seaside you can sit silently on the beach, hearing the sound of the waves, feeling the breeze on your face — keep hearing and feeling, without thinking, until you and the beach, the ocean and the wind become one.

It doesn't matter where you are, you can take time out to meditate. However, mornings and evenings are the best times. Once you start your meditation regime you will find enormous benefits, on both a physical and a spiritual level.

*See also Stress and Tension.*

# Memory Loss

Forgetfulness can affect all age groups. Lapses of concentration can account for much of this. Unfortunately, there is no magic cure for memory loss.

Fortifying the brain with vitamins, minerals and herbs may help any deterioration and enable those people experiencing the beginning of a decline in their cognitive functions to maintain a normal life. Certain vitamins, minerals and micro-nutrients do seem to have a significant effect on the function of the brain: in particular, vitamins C and E, potassium, selenium and zinc. These vitamins and minerals can easily be obtained as supplements, and if taken daily they may be beneficial.

Herbs such as rosemary and sage are steeped in tradition for improving memory, and both herbs do seem to have the ability to promote the supply of blood and oxygen to the brain. Ginkgo (*Ginkgo biloba*), an ancient Chinese herb which enjoys a similar reputation, has been credited with helping both short-term memory and slowing of the ageing process. Ginkgo supplies the brain with glucose, its principal source of energy. All three herbs can be taken as a herbal tea 3–4 times a day, or as needed.

# Menopause

Many women are a little afraid of the approach of menopause, and see it as the beginning of a decline in the quality of their life. There is hormone replacement therapy, but the experts have yet to agree as to what physiological problems may result from it. HRT is a matter of individual choice.

Good nutrition, including plenty of raw fruit and vegetables, sufficient vitamin intake, the use of cold-pressed cooking oils and a supplement of evening primrose oil will all be beneficial. Natural herbal supplements specifically formulated for menopause can also be taken. Exclude stimulants from your diet, especially tea, coffee and alcohol; drink non-addictive herbal teas instead.

Including ginseng in your diet will give you a natural source of oestrogen. Check with your health practitioner first, since ginseng is a natural steroid. Headaches, migraine, dizziness and nausea can be treated by taking 1 small glass of fresh cucumber juice a day.

Including cypress, geranium or sage oil in your bath or in a daily massage oil will help relieve circulatory problems, hot flushes, day and night sweats and water retention. Blend in a 9:16:5 ratio with 30 ml of almond oil, and store in an airtight, amber-coloured glass bottle.

When massaging, always massage in the direction of the heart: from the feet to the thighs and from the hands to the shoulders. If your whole body is affected, have someone massage both the front and back of your torso, and use no more than 1 teaspoon of oil. This should be done daily, in conjunction with a warm, relaxing bath. Add 10 drops of the same oil blend to hot bathwater once it has settled.

# Menstrual Problems

No two women are alike in the way their monthly period affects them. For many it is accompanied by unpleasant side effects, such as uterine cramp, muscular and abdominal pain, water retention, sore breasts, headaches, fatigue, irritability and depression. Some women suffer from profuse menstruation, while others have a scanty menstrual flow. If your state of health is good there is usually no need to concern yourself about a scanty period. However, it is advisable to include the following in your diet: fresh grated beetroot, barley, green beans, strawberries, lettuce, brown rice and soya beans. Diet will also assist women who are prone to a heavy period — the following should be eaten on a regular basis: carrots, lentils, parsley, ginger and fresh pineapple. Fibre is also important for all menstrual problems — include buckwheat, pulses and oats in your diet, and avoid bread.

Vegetables to help combat water retention are cucumber, watermelon, celery, asparagus and globe artichokes. Watermelon, when in season, is one of the most effective diuretic fruits. Diuretic herbs that are beneficial include dandelion leaves, dandelion roots (made into a coffee substitute, available from health food stores) and parsley. Take the herbs as a tea 2–3 times a day. A low-salt diet is also helpful.

If you think you retain too much fluid, get your health practitioner to check out your heart and kidneys before you try any treatment.

Certain essentials oils are also useful in easing the various problems and alleviating discomfort. However, with conditions such as continuous water retention, pain and irritability and other long-term symptoms, medical attention is essential.

Essential oils are delightful to use in any body preparation, and quite apart from their therapeutic qualities, their marvellous fragrance will leave you feeling special.

When using essential oils to help relieve menstrual problems, use them in moderation and only as a crutch. They can be applied as a body rub or added to your bath. Do not attempt to use them internally.

Oils to use on their own or in combination are rose, oregano, marjoram, melissa, geranium, nutmeg, bergamot, clary sage, rosemary, cypress, chamomile and myrrh. For a body rub, add 30 drops of essential oil to 30 ml of almond oil and store in an airtight, amber-coloured glass bottle. You can add 1 teaspoon of the body lotion to a warm bath or add 8–10 drops of neat essential oil to your bath each day.

To apply the body rub, adopt self-massage techniques (*see Massage [Self-Body Massage]*). Concentrate only on the abdomen, hips and lower back, extending down between the buttocks but keeping well clear of the anus.

The following blends are general formulas, and may not suit every individual.

### Massage Oil Blend for
### Abdominal Pain and Cramp

*30 ml almond oil*
*9 drops cypress essential oil*
*9 drops clary sage essential oil*
*12 drops chamomile essential oil*

Relief from cramping can be obtained
by rubbing an oregano oil blend
into the lower parts of the body.
In addition, linseed tea, taken as
needed, can give relief from the
pain. To make the tea, add 2
tablespoons of linseeds to 750
ml of boiling water. Add a
pinch of cinnamon, the juice
of ½ lemon and 1 teaspoon of brown
sugar. Simmer over a gentle heat for about
20 minutes, and strain before use.

### Severe menstrual pain

For severe menstrual pain, take 15 drops of spirit of balm in a glass of
water every ½ hour.

Spirit of balm is made from the tangy lemon-scented leaves of *Melissa
officinalis* (lemon balm). It grows quickly from seed, is self-seeding, and
will grow almost anywhere. You can make your own spirit of balm
blend as follows:

*1 cup tightly packed fresh lemon balm leaves*
*750 ml high-proof vodka*
*750 ml distilled water*

Put all the ingredients in a glass jar, seal with an airtight lid and leave
in a warm place for several days. Strain the mixture, drip through
coffee filter paper and store in an airtight glass bottle. Use as
directed above.

## PRE-MENSTRUAL TENSION

If you suffer pre-menstrual tension, eat plenty of green leafy vegetables, including fresh young dandelion leaves if you can, and a breakfast of grapefruit and plums or pears. Use any of the following essential oils in a body rub and/or added to your bath: rose, bergamot, geranium, clary sage, cypress, nutmeg and chamomile.

A suggested oil blend is:

*30 ml almond oil*
*9 drops chamomile essential oil*
*9 drops bergamot essential oil*
*12 drops rose essential oil*

*See also Chamomile, Headache, Pre-Menstrual Headache.*

# Mental Fatigue

When your concentration is flagging, you will find that inhaling a few drops of basil and bergamot oil on a handkerchief will help.

*See also Exercise, Fatigue, Revitalisation, Stress and Tension.*

# Midges

*See Insect Bite Itch, Stings and Bites.*

# Migraine Headache

The herb feverfew (*Tanacetum parthenium*) is extremely good for preventing migraine headaches and alleviating the pain and associated discomfort. As a preventive measure, eat 3 leaves of the fresh herb a day in a sandwich, or take feverfew capsules (available from health food stores), or drink feverfew tea.

*See Headache (Migraine Headaches).*

# Milk Thistle

This thorny, weed-like herb was once popular in Germany in the treatment of jaundice and biliary complaints. Nowadays, it is also gaining prominence as a healing tonic for the liver. Silymarin, the active ingredient in milk thistle (*Silybum marianum*), is considered a powerful antioxidant that aids in the prevention of free radical damage to the liver. It also helps the liver detoxify alcohol and fatty foods.

Tablets and capsules are available from health food stores.

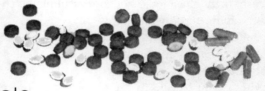

# Minerals

Minerals control the body's chemical balance, and an adequate intake is necessary if you are to achieve the ideal state of physical equilibrium. The mineral requirements of your body differ from time to time, and it is therefore important to maintain a balanced intake of correct foodstuffs to keep your body functioning in peak condition.

*See separate listings for Calcium, Chlorine, Iodine, Iron, Magnesium, Phosphorus, Potassium, Silicon, Sodium, Sulphur, Trace Minerals, Zinc.*

# Mineral Deficiencies

Take bran internally. Put 2 tablespoons of bran into a saucepan and pour 500 ml of boiling water over it. Bring to the boil and simmer over a low heat for about 15 minutes, then cool and strain. Drink 1 cupful 3–5 times a day, as required.

*See also Calcium, Chlorine, Iodine, Iron, Magnesium, Phosphorus, Potassium, Silicon, Sodium, Sulphur, Trace Minerals, Zinc.*

# Mites

Usually, mites are too small to be seen with the naked eye. An infestation can be a continual source of irritation, and can result in a rash, or even dermatitis.

Most mites can be washed off with some very hot soapy water. First, soak in a hot bath to which you have added 10 ml each of eucalyptus oil and lavender oil. Scrub yourself thoroughly with a bristly brush, then take a long, hot shower immediately after your bath, soaping and rinsing thoroughly.

If the mites don't respond to the soap-and-water treatment, seek professional help to determine exactly what sort of mite infestation you have.

Other things you can do to get rid of mites are to air carpets, mats, cushions and lounge covers for several days. Place them in a plastic bag with a few sprigs of lavender and leave them outside in the sun, or have them dry-cleaned. Do likewise with bed linen (after thoroughly vacuuming the floors).

# Mosquito Bite

*See Insect Bite Itch, Stings and Bites.*

# Mouth

## INFLAMED AND SORE GUMS

Prepare a soothing lotion by diluting 6 drops of myrrh essential oil and 4 drops of lavender essential oil in 40 ml of aloe vera juice. Store in an airtight, amber-coloured glass bottle. Apply after using the gingivitis gargle below, smoothing a little of the lotion on inflamed and sore gums.

## GINGIVITIS

Use the following mouthwash as required: dilute 2 drops each of lemon and eucalyptus oil and 1 drop of lavender oil in 1 teaspoon of vodka. Blend the mixture with 1 cup of warm water, then rinse your mouth, but do not swallow. Any excess mouthwash can be kept in the refrigerator. Warm before using.

## GUM BOILS

Dilute 2 drops of chamomile essential oil and 1 drop of thyme essential oil with 20 ml of aloe vera juice. Dab a little on boils and smooth around ulcerated areas 2–3 times a day. Store the mixture in an airtight, amber-coloured glass bottle away from direct heat and sunlight.

## MOUTH ULCERS

Mouth ulcers are caused by a minor viral infection and will usually respond to a mouthwash and ointment. However, persistent ulcers or acute problems should be referred immediately to your health practitioner.

### *Mouthwash*

*1 drop peppermint essential oil*
*1 drop geranium essential oil*
*1 drop thyme essential oil*
*2 drops lemon essential oil*
*5 ml brandy*
*250 ml distilled water*

Dilute the essential oils in the brandy and then mix thoroughly with the water. Swish around inside your mouth several times but do not swallow.

### *Aloe Vera Ointment*

*2 drops chamomile essential oil*
*1 drop thyme essential oil*
*20 ml aloe vera juice (available from health food stores)*

Blend the oils thoroughly with the aloe vera juice and store in the
refrigerator in an airtight, amber-coloured glass bottle.
Use within 3 days — if the mixture begins to smell rancid,
discard it immediately and make a new batch. Smooth a
little of the ointment around the ulcerated area after using
the mouthwash.

*See also Oral Hygiene.*

## PYORRHOEA

This condition is characterised by recession of the gums and loose
teeth. An immediate first aid treatment is to rub a little eucalyptus
oil into your gums. To heal your gums and prevent further
damage, include plenty of natural raw food in your diet.

*See Oral Hygiene (Healthy Gums).*
*See also Bad Breath, Sage, Thyme.*

# Muscle Spasms

Spasmed muscles are usually the result of prolonged stress, caused
by intense physical or emotional tension over time. Muscles are
worked beyond their limits, resulting in a lack of electrolytes in
the blood.

This type of stress, which is usually manifested in our necks,
can be caused by emotional problems at work or home. The
inability to express our emotional state results in tight or stressed
muscles. The neck muscles are more often than not the muscles
where this stress is felt.

Over a prolonged period stress of this nature restricts blood
supply to the muscles, which then become so starved of nutrients

and oxygen that they are unable to return to their former relaxed state. At this stage the spasm is chronic and becomes painful. If this condition persists, it will cause further emotional stress, and increased pain and discomfort, until the spasm is relieved.

Spasmed muscles are sometimes not painful to begin with, but they are noticed as the inability to move the neck or a limb through its full range of movement increases.

Stiffness of the neck is not just a physical condition; it is also reflected in mental inflexibility. It is difficult to think creatively and be able to consider someone else's point of view objectively. A stiff and inflexible neck leads to stiff and inflexible thinking.

The muscle most often spasmed in the neck is the trapezius: the large muscle on top of the shoulder, stretching from the base of the neck out to the arm socket. However, a good massage will quickly relieved stressed neck muscles.

## SELF-MASSAGE TECHNIQUE

Place a hand on the top of the opposite trapezius muscle, with your fingers resting on the top of your back and your thumb resting just under your collarbone. Knead the tissue gently by working the fingers together in a circular motion from your shoulder along the trapezius to the base of your skull, lifting your thumb from beneath your collarbone as your fingers reach your neck, and continuing to work with your fingers. The thumb supports your hand from the front while your fingers do the work.

Give yourself this massage just after a warm shower or bath, or at work while you are having a break, or whenever you need to alleviate tension and stress.

# Muscular Aches and Pains

Dissolve ½ cup of bicarbonate of soda in a hot bath and soak in it. Follow this with a massage of the painful and aching areas with the following ointment: 2 crushed garlic cloves mixed well with a 100 g raw petroleum jelly. Store in an airtight jar.

Six drops each of eucalyptus and lavender oil mixed together and massaged into the painful area will also help. I have found this an excellent remedy to relieve stiffness and soreness associated with working in the garden.

## MUSCULAR STRAIN

*See Sprains and Strains.*

## MUSCULAR CRAMP

Muscular cramps can be eased by the following herbal tea.

*1 teaspoon powdered cinnamon*
*1/2 teaspoon powdered cardamom*
*1/4 teaspoon powdered nutmeg*

Add all the ingredients to a ceramic cup of boiling water, stir until thoroughly mixed, cover, and infuse for 5 minutes. Sip the tea while it is still warm.

## TIGHT MUSCLES

For a warming, soothing liniment that helps loosen muscles and gets them ready for sport, mix eucalyptus or rosemary oil, a drop at a time, with almond oil, ensuring that the mixture remains strongly scented, and massage into your muscles until you feel a warm glow.

*See also Aching Joints and Muscles, Aromatic Shower, Bathing, Chamomile, Joints (Painful), Lavender, Massage, Sprains and Strains, Thyme.*

# N

## Nails

*See Hands (Fingernails).*

## Nappy Rash

Garlic water or oil applied externally will help to soothe irritation. *See Yeast Infection.*

Alternatively, bathe the affected area with Chamomile Nappy Wash whenever the nappy is changed.

### Chamomile Nappy Wash

*1 cup dried chamomile flowers*
*1 cup dried elder flowers*

Put the herbs in a ceramic bowl, add sufficient boiling water to cover by about 2 cm, cover the bowl and leave to infuse overnight. Next day, strain through clean muslin cloth, squeezing all liquid from the herbs. Store in a sterilised, airtight bottle in the refrigerator for no longer than 7 days. If the lotion begins to smell unpleasant any earlier, discard it and make a fresh batch.

*See also Garlic.*

## Nasal Congestion

Inhalation is particularly useful when suffering from a head cold, sinusitis or nasal congestion. Steaming offers an effective and direct method of treating respiratory and sinus problems. Oils ideal for vaporising are peppermint, eucalyptus and tea-tree. Peppermint and eucalyptus contain menthol and eucalyptol respectively, and have a cooling effect on tissues and tired muscles. Other oils will smooth out that crumpled look and restore tone to facial muscles.

The action of steam is twofold: internal as well as external. Essences in the vapour are absorbed through the delicate membrane of the nasal passages and through exposed skin, as in a facial massage.

To make your own vaporiser, half fill a ceramic bowl with boiling water, add 5 drops of oil, hold your face about 30 cm away and cover your head with a towel large enough to form a tent. Do not allow the vapour to escape. You should not steam your face for any longer than 10 minutes, and no more than 3 times a day. People with heart and blood pressure problems, asthma or other breathing difficulties, broken skin or visible, dilated red veins should avoid using steam inhalations, unless otherwise directed by their health practitioner.

An effective head-clearing inhalation to use for colds and flu is to blend 2 drops each of eucalyptus and rosemary oil, 1 drop of lavender oil or 2 drops each of tea-tree and sandalwood oil and 1 drop of eucalyptus oil. For sinusitis, blend 2 drops each of peppermint, eucalyptus and rosemary oil, or 2 drops each of basil, eucalyptus, lavender and peppermint oil.

When at work or travelling, a portable inhalant is an ideal treatment. Add 5–8 drops of essential oil to a handkerchief or tissue and take 4 deep breaths, then inhale the scent whenever needed. When the handkerchief is not in use, you should place it against your breastbone, where it will continue to work. It can also be placed beside your pillow at night to facilitate easier breathing.

*See also Allergies, Colds, Hay Fever, Sinusitis, Vinaigrette.*

# Nausea

Freshly grated ginger or powdered cinnamon infused with hot water, or sprinkled in other herbal teas, can be taken as required to relieve the symptoms of nausea and vomiting.

Clove tea is another excellent remedy for allaying nausea and vomiting, while at the same time stimulating the digestive system. Add 10 cloves to a ceramic cup, pour 250 ml of boiling water over them, cover and infuse for 10 minutes. Reheat if required and take as necessary.

# Nervous Tension

The herb valerian is a very powerful natural sedative and tranquilliser; unlike its synthetic counterpart, it is not habit forming. Take it as a cold tea to relieve nervous tension, insomnia and restlessness.

The tea is made by infusing the dried root in boiling water and allowing to stand for 12 hours. The tea is slightly bitter — the taste can be improved by the addition of honey. Drink no more than 3 cups in any one day.

*See also Insomnia, Sleep.*

# Nettle

Depending upon your point of view, a stinging nettle is either a very useful plant or an unattractive weed that stings when touched. With care, the nettle can be enjoyed and employed, as the leaves lose their sting when they are boiled or dried.

Every part of the plant — leaf, root and seed — is rich in vitamins, iron, protein, silicic acid, nitrogen, chlorophyll and other trace elements. They provide a nutritional, staple green that can be enjoyed in summer salads or cooked like spinach.

### *Nettle Soup*

*1 handful young nettle leaves*
*2 tablespoons tofu*
*400 g potatoes*
*1 onion, chopped*
*1 litre stock*
*soya milk*

Wearing rubber gloves, cut nettle stalks and select the youngest and greenest leaves. Cook in a saucepan with half the tofu. No extra liquid is needed. Fry the potatoes, and onion with the remaining tofu until golden in colour. Add the nettle leaves and tofu and stir together. Pour in the stock and cook gently for 20–30 minutes, or until tender. Process in a blender with a little soya milk, to make the soup creamy.

## NETTLE HAIR CONDITIONING LOTION

This conditioning lotion is reputed to prevent falling hair, stimulate growth and leave your hair shiny and healthy.

Place a handful of fresh young nettle leaves into an enamel or stainless steel saucepan and cover with almond oil. Bring to just below boiling and simmer until the herbs are crisp. Allow to cool, strain, add a few drops of rosemary oil until it is just fragrant, store in a bottle and seal tightly.

Massage into the scalp 2–3 times a week, after washing your hair.

*See also Hair.*

# Nettle Rash

Apply 1–2 drops of eucalyptus oil to the affected area. Then make up the following mixture and spread it over the rash: dissolve 5 drops each of lavender and eucalyptus oil in 1 tablespoon of aloe vera juice.

Take a warm bath, to which has been added ¼ cup of Epsom salts and 4 drops of chamomile oil.

*See also Itchiness, Rashes, Skin Irritations.*

# Neuralgia

Numb the area with ice first, then use any of the following treatments:

◗ Cut wedges of lemon and rub onto the painful area.

- Place hot chamomile tea bags against the painful area. Replace frequently with fresh, hot tea bags.
- During the day drink a cup of celery tea as needed for the relief of pain.
- Relieve inflammation by gently massaging the area with the following massage oil: dissolve 5 drops each of lavender and chamomile oil and 2 drops of rosemary oil in 10 ml of almond oil.

*See also Chamomile.*

# Nightmares

Avoid eating acid or hard-to-digest foods as a night snack. Maintain regular mealtime habits, to enable your digestive system to sleep when the rest of your body sleeps.

Drink a cup of chamomile or hops tea before retiring.

# Nits

*See Head Lice.*

# Nosebleeds

A bloody nose will stop within seconds if you put a bit of calendula ointment up the offending nostril. A wad of rolled-up yarrow leaf inserted into the nostril is also effective.

If you suffer continually from nosebleeds, it's more than likely that you lack iron — you may need to consider a supplement. Speak to your health practitioner first, as some iron supplements can lead to constipation.

## FIRST AID TREATMENT FOR A NOSEBLEED

- Gently blow your nose, then sit upright and lean your head slightly forward. Don't lean your head back — the blood will run down your throat.

- Pinch both nostrils below the bridge between your thumb and forefinger, and, while breathing through your mouth, hold your nose firmly for up to 10 minutes. This will allow the blood vessels to repair themselves and stop the bleeding.
- Once bleeding has stopped, under no circumstances blow your nose or bend over for at least 2 hours.

# Nutrition

To get healthy or to remain healthy, our bodies need fuel in the form of food. What we eat determines what happens to our bodies. It is essential, therefore, that we eat the correct foods, in the correct proportions, from all the food groups: carbohydrates (including fibre), protein and fats. We also need a correct balance of vitamins, minerals, trace elements and water.

## CARBOHYDRATES

Carbohydrates are divided into 3 main groups — complex carbohydrates, sugars and fibre. They are the fuel that provides our bodies with the get-up-and-go we need. Dietary fibre is also a carbohydrate, commonly known as 'roughage'.

## COMPLEX CARBOHYDRATES (STARCHES)

Bread, cereals, fruit, legumes and vegetables are in this group. When digested, complex carbohydrates are converted into glucose. However, if the glucose is not required immediately by the body it is stored in the liver as glycogen. This provides an energy reserve.

Body energy requirements are far better taken from complex carbohydrates than from simple sugars. Energy is released more slowly and will therefore last longer.

Complex carbohydrates also contain fibre, protein, vitamins and minerals, all of which are lacking in sugar.

## SUGARS

The digestive process breaks sugars down so that they are absorbed into the bloodstream as glucose, which is the basal fuel for the brain.

Sugars fall into the following groups:

- sucrose — mainly from sugar cane
- glucose — sweet fruits, honey and corn
- fructose — ripe fruits, honey and some vegetables
- maltose — grains such as barley and wheat
- lactose — only from milk.

## REFINED SUGAR

Beware of sugar, especially refined white sugar. It contains nothing but empty, fattening, tooth-rotting calories. An excessive intake of refined sugar has been blamed for causing increased tooth plaque, tooth decay and anaemia, kidney lesions, dermatitis, weight gain, and blood pressure and heart problems.

Refined sugar, which is found in a large number of the foods we buy and consume, can easily replace lost energy — it is quickly digested, converted into glucose, and passed into the bloodstream. The downside of relying on refined sugars for an 'energy fix' is that, in some cases, the increased insulin produced by the pancreas can actually lower the blood sugar to below its previous level. This will leave you feeling far more tired, hungry and depressed than you were previously.

It is far better to obtain that 'energy fix' from the sugars that occur naturally in fruit and vegetables. Although its conversion to glucose and glycogen is slower, the energy lasts longer, without the associated 'low' that is experienced from refined sugar consumption.

Remember, look for the 'hidden' sugar when doing your grocery shopping, or, for that matter, when purchasing any packaged food. Labels can be very misleading, and many products will lead you to believe that they are sugar-free by using the following names: lactose, glucose, maltose, levulose, invertase, corn syrup, maple syrup, dextrose, fructose and sucrose. If any of these names are on the label, you will know that sugar has been added.

## FIBRE

Dietary fibre is a carbohydrate made up of the material which forms the cell walls of plants. There are 2 types of fibre: insoluble fibre, such as wheat bran, and soluble fibre, such as fruits and legumes. Insoluble fibre cannot be digested by body enzymes, so it passes through the body as roughage. Soluble fibre is easily digested; it is processed by useful bacteria and produces valuable acids.

Insoluble fibre is essential for a properly functioning bowel. It holds water and shortens the time taken for food waste to leave the body. Lack of sufficient insoluble fibre in your diet will cause constipation.

Soluble fibre helps control blood sugar and cholesterol levels. Research has shown that lack of fibre in the human diet may lead to such conditions as piles, obesity, diverticulitis, and even bowel cancer. It is important, therefore, to get enough fibre by maintaining a well-balanced diet, not to get your fibre by simply sprinkling large amounts of raw bran over your breakfast cereal. This can actually have a detrimental effect on the body — more than 2 tablespoons a day could irritate your oesophagus, and nutritional deficiencies could also occur due to excessive nutrient loss through bowel movements.

The best way to start the day, and to ensure that you receive an adequate supply of both types of fibre, is to have a good breakfast of whole cereals, then a snack of washed, unpeeled fruit mid-morning and mid-afternoon, and salads and raw, or slightly cooked, vegetables with your lunch and evening meal. Eat wholemeal bread, rice and pastas instead of the refined varieties, and include plenty of legumes, nuts and dried fruits in your diet. Include at least 40–50 g of fibre a day — do this and you will feel healthy, vibrant and vital. Remember, highly refined carbohydrates lose many essential nutrients, along with fibre, during their processing, whereas unrefined carbohydrates retain fibre, vitamins and minerals.

# O

## Oats

*See Eating for Health and Energy.*

## Obesity

In our modern society obesity has become more and more common. Busy lives and a fast pace, coupled with ready-in-a-minute takeaway food, have left us wanting. Yet, of all the human diseases, obesity is the least chronic and the easiest to overcome. It's as simple as replacing 'will power' with 'won't power'.

Obesity is usually the result of the amount and nature of the food one eats. When the diet includes a significant amount of fresh raw fruits and vegetables, the chances of becoming overweight are rare, if not nil. If you eliminate junk food altogether, do not eat more food than your body requires, and exercise regularly, obesity will not be a problem for you. This may seem an oversimplification, but the fact remains that overweight people do eat more food than necessary, and that their food is invariably composed of cooked and processed non-nutritive substances.

There are no miracle diets, or magic weight loss pills — but you can take a sensible approach to eating, maintain a positive mental attitude and take pride in your appearance. For those of you who feel that making fresh raw fruits and vegetables the mainstay (80 per cent) of your diet is not possible, and who don't wish to give up meat or dairy foods, the following tips may be of help.

Make sure you eat breakfast, lunch and dinner. Don't skip meals — you will just get hungry, and you will more than likely eat too much at the next meal.

Base your diet on breads and grain-based foods, fruit and vegetables, lean meats, low-fat dairy foods, lean poultry, fish and legumes. If you feel you must include cheese, include only a small portion each week, and ensure that it is low-fat. Better still, replace it with a cheese substitute, such as tofu. Include no more than 2 eggs each week, if you must have them.

Avoid too much fat (butter, margarine, oil, cream, salad dressing), sugar, salt and alcohol. Take advantage of the low-kilojoule products now available — sugar-free soft drinks, cordials, low-kilojoule jellies, oil-free salad dressings. And drink plenty of water.

Accept the fact that you may break your diet from time to time. Don't use this an excuse to binge; just get yourself back on track. Bingeing will only make you feel depressed, and will quickly lead to eating too much food again, especially sweet substances.

If you do crave sweet foods occasionally, direct these cravings to fresh fruit.

Cut back, or eliminate completely, your alcohol intake. Alcohol itself does not contain fat, but it is still a high source of kilojoules, following closely behind fat at 29 kilojoules per g.

Be realistic about your achievements and consult with your health practitioner before embarking on any dietary changes.

---

*See also Dietary Substitutes, Eating for Health and Energy.*

# Onion

The onion is one of the most famous food and medicinal plants of history. It is highly nutritious, an excellent disinfectant, a natural antibiotic, and is rich in vitamin B1. A regular intake of onion will ensure that your nervous system remains healthy.

Taken as a syrup, it will aid in digestion and will help relieve the miseries of a cold. A bowl of onion soup will help bring out a fever and restore lost energy.

### Onion Syrup

*1 large grated onion*
*2 tablespoons honey*
*1 bottle white wine*

Put all the ingredients in a ceramic bowl. Cover and allow to steep for
2 weeks, making sure to stir the mixture morning and night. Strain
through sterile muslin and store in an airtight glass bottle.
Take 1 tablespoon morning and night when needed.

### Onion Soup

*2 medium-sized onions*
*2 medium-sized potatoes*
*50 g butter*
*1 garlic clove, crushed*
*1 litre stock*
*125 ml light milk*
*parsley, basil and thyme*

Slice the onions and potatoes. Melt the butter in a pan with a heavy
base and add the potatoes, onions and crushed garlic. Cook over a low
heat, stirring from time to time. Mix in the stock, bring to the boil, then
simmer for about 20 minutes, by which time the vegetables will be
tender. Stir in the milk, season with herbs and reheat to simmering point.
Eat as is or process in a blender first.

# Oral Hygiene

Looking after your gums and teeth is as important as caring for
the rest of your body. Correct oral hygiene means a healthy mouth
and sweet breath. If plaque isn't removed daily, it eventually builds
up, causing gum disease — inflammation, swelling and bleeding
are the first signs of gingivitis.

Some simple rules to follow, which will help to keep your teeth
in top condition, are:

▶ Brush and floss your teeth at least twice a day.
▶ Brush or rinse your mouth after each snack.

- Have a dental check-up twice a year.
- Maintain a well-balanced diet, including herbs that help keep teeth healthy and strong. Healthy teeth need peak nutrition — especially the minerals, calcium, magnesium and phosphorus, and the trace elements.

## Herbs which provide these elements:

CALCIUM

alfalfa, chamomile, dandelion, nettle, parsley and strawberry (fruit)

MAGNESIUM

alfalfa, cayenne, dandelion and peppermint

PHOSPHORUS

alfalfa, caraway, cayenne, chickweed, dandelion, garlic, parsley and watercress

TRACE MINERALS

alfalfa and kelp (seaweed)

## Natural food sources for these elements:

CALCIUM

almonds, Brazil nuts, cheese, yogurt, molasses, salmon, sardines, prawns, soya beans, tofu, sunflower seeds, leafy green vegetables, wheat germ and a balanced intake of dairy products

MAGNESIUM

almonds and other nuts, fish, prawns, leafy green vegetables, molasses, soya beans, sunflower seeds and wheat germ

PHOSPHORUS

whole grains, beans, nuts, wheat germ, oatmeal, pumpkin seeds, lentils, sunflower seeds, sesame seeds, soya beans, sprouted seeds, brown rice, kelp, garlic, mushrooms, sweet corn, sweet potato, dried peaches and apricots, and a balanced intake of dairy products

## CLEAN YOUR TEETH CORRECTLY

Hold the bristles of your brush at a 45° angle to your gum, then move the brush in tiny circles. Clean the inside and outside of your front and back teeth as well as the biting surfaces of all your lower and upper teeth.

## HEALTHY GUMS

Brushing your gums is just as important as brushing your teeth. Angle your brush to reach under the gum margin and gently massage. When you have finished, rinse out your mouth with water, then remove any plaque between your teeth with dental floss. Next, rub fresh sage leaves over your teeth and gums; this will leave your mouth feeling cleansed, and will help whiten your teeth and strengthen your gums.

## THE NATURAL WAY TO CLEAN TEETH

Healthy teeth are not only produced by the use of toothpastes, which quite often promise all sorts of amazing things. Your teeth and gums can be kept in tiptop condition if you clean them with herbs and other natural, safe ingredients.

A quick and simple tooth powder can be made by combining salt and bicarbonate of soda. Thoroughly mix together 2 tablespoons of fine sea salt and 3 tablespoons of bicarbonate of soda. Store in a dry, airtight jar. To use, shake a little of the mixture into your hand and pick it up with a damp toothbrush.

To make a herbal tooth powder mix 15 g of fresh sage leaves and 10 g of fresh peppermint leaves with 20 g of coarse sea salt. Spread this out on a baking tray, then place in a preheated oven (150°C) for 20 minutes, or until the herbs are crisp and dry. Reduce the dried herbs to a powder by rubbing them through a fine wire sieve. Store in a dry, airtight jar.

To use your tooth powder, shake a little of the mixture into your hand and pick it up with a damp toothbrush.

## MOUTHWASH

To keep your breath sweet and your mouth tasting fresh, try this herbal mouthwash. Place 2 teaspoons of dried sage and 1 teaspoon each of dried peppermint and rosemary in a ceramic bowl and cover with 2 cups of boiling water. Add ½ cup of brandy or cider vinegar, cover the bowl and steep for 2 hours. Strain through fine muslin and then drip through coffee filter paper. Store in a tightly sealed bottle.

Use the mouthwash as a soothing gargle or as a refreshing rinse as needed.

*See also Bad Breath, Mouth, Sage, Thyme*

# Oregano

Taken as a tea, oregano will expel flatulence, induce perspiration, ease cramps and griping pains, relieve painful menstruation, asthma and catarrh of the air passages. It will help to soothe a nagging cough. When the oil is rubbed into the abdomen it will relieve menstrual pain and cramping. The essential oil can also be used as a rub in the treatment of bruises, sprains and muscular pain.

Oregano (*Origanum vulgare*) will readily grow in the home garden. The dried herb and essential oil are available from health food stores.

# Osteoporosis

*See Exercise.*

# Overindulgence

Regardless of good intentions, it happens every Christmas. We swear that we won't overindulge in all those tempting goodies, yet, somehow, many of us still succumb.

There is no way to miraculously dissolve away all that excess food, but we can use herbs and essential oils to relieve the associated discomfort. Better still, be realistic and prepare yourself for the inevitable.

Chamomile tea is excellent for calming down an overworked stomach; spearmint tea aids digestion and helps dispel stomach gas. A mixture of equal parts peppermint, lemon balm and lemon verbena tea can be drunk after a heavy meal to aid digestion. Add 1 teaspoon of dried herb (or 1 teaspoon of a mixture of them) to a ceramic cup, pour in hot water, infuse for 3 minutes, and strain into another cup. Adjust to taste with honey (or lemon juice, if preferred).

Another simple tea to aid digestion can be made using one of the following: lemon oil, ginger oil or peppermint oil. Put 1 or 2 drops of your chosen oil and a teaspoon of honey into a mug, pour in boiling water, stir until dissolved, and sip slowly.

Overindulgence in alcohol leads to dehydration, and results in those miserable sensations commonly called a hangover. To a greater or lesser degree the body is having to cope with poisoning.

Beers and wines vary enormously in their chemical content: some are classed as being organic — their ingredients were cultivated without chemicals, and no chemicals were added in their processing. Others, however, are almost pure chemical cocktails. Drinking good-quality organic beverages lessens the effects of hangovers in the short term and, in the longer term, will do less damage to your liver.

Other preventive measures against hangover include drinking plenty of water before you drink alcohol, or in between alcoholic drinks. This slows down the alcohol absorption rate and allows your body to cope better. Drinking plenty of water after the party is over will help flush the toxins from your body. Before going to sleep, take around 1000 mg of vitamin C, but do not take any more than this (more than 1000 mg could cause diarrhoea). Avoid drinking black coffee — this will only make things worse.

The best antidote for a hangover and indigestion, however, is moderation. Drink and eat sensibly, and your body will thank you.

*See also Acidity, Hangover, Indigestion, Medicinal Food, Stomach, Thyme.*

# P

## Pain Relief

*See specific listing for ailment, and also Aches and Pains, Aching
Joints and Muscles, Aromatic Shower, Bathing, Chamomile,
Compresses, Feverfew, Flatulence, Garlic (Garlic Ointment),
Herbal Teas (Alfalfa, Lemon Balm), Lavender, Massage,
Menstrual Problems, Muscular Aches and Pains, Neuralgia,
Oregano, Tea-Tree Oil, Thyme, Valerian, Witch Hazel Ointment.*

## Parsley

This highly nutritious herb (*Petroselinum crispum*) is rich in
organic iron, potassium, silicon and magnesium, and contains
vitamins A, B and C as well as other trace elements. Eaten
regularly, it is a helpful remedy for anaemic conditions and
stimulates the appetite and digestive juices. Taken as a tea it has a
cleansing effect, acts as an overall tonic, and assists the bladder,
kidneys and liver. Cooled, it is an excellent lotion for reducing
puffiness around the eyes. Parsley's high nutritive value helps in
arthritic pain, will bring down a fever, and dry up mother's milk
after childbirth. Chewing the fresh leaf will sweeten the breath,
especially after eating garlic; when the leaves are bruised and
steeped in vinegar and placed next to the breasts, they will relieve
swelling.

Parsley can easily be grown in the home garden.

## Peptic Ulcer

*See Ulcers.*

# Phosphorus

Phosphorus helps the nervous system remain healthy and at peak performance. It has a tonic effect on the circulation and is essential for maintaining healthy skin, hair and fingernails. In combination with calcium it tends to produce a neutral body environment and a state of balance.

The best sources of phosphorus are seeds and grain foods; these should be included in your diet every day. Natural sources are alfalfa, apricots (dried), beans, brown rice, dandelion, garlic, kelp, lentils, mushrooms, nuts, oatmeal, parsley, peaches (dried), pumpkin seeds, sesame seeds, soya beans, sprouted seeds, sunflower seeds, sweet corn, sweet potato, watercress, wheat germ and dairy products.

# Pimples

*See Acne.*

# Plant Stings

*See Stings and Bites.*

# Potassium

Along with sodium, potassium helps regulate the balance of body fluid. The liver is the primary place of potassium metabolism, where glycogen is formed and stored. Potassium also regulates muscle function, and therefore helps the heart and ensures good muscle tone and good muscular energy and response.

Potassium-rich foods should be eaten regularly by people suffering from arthritis and rheumatism. Because its biochemical reaction is alkaline, potassium helps balance acid accumulations in the body.

Natural sources of potassium are avocado, apricots (dried), bananas (dried), beans (all dried varieties), beetroot, cabbage, cauliflower, celery, chickpeas, coconut meat, cucumber, dandelion greens, horseradish, legumes, lettuce, parsley, peaches (fresh), rice bran, radish, seaweed (edible types — agar, dulse, kelp, Irish moss), sesame seeds, sunflower seeds, tomato, watercress, wheat bran and wheat germ.

# Pregnancy

For many women, pregnancy causes changes and upheavals in the body that result in considerable discomfort and stress. Minor problems such as backache, swollen legs, reversal of skin condition (oily to dry or vice versa), lack of skin tone, morning sickness and insomnia can be relieved by the use of essential oils, plus moderate exercise and dietary modification.

Include plenty of fresh fruit and vegetables (in particular broad beans, climbing and dwarf beans and peas), wholemeal cereal products, poultry and fish in your diet. Avoid red meat as much as possible — completely abstain from it if you can. Exercise daily by walking and/or swimming until it no longer feels comfortable. Only undertake an exercise programme after consultation with your health practitioner.

## BACKACHE AND SWOLLEN LEGS

Among the lesser joys of pregnancy are backache, swollen legs and tiredness.

The uplifting qualities of essential oils will help ease the aches and lethargy, soothe the spirits and put the world back in perspective. Add them to a warm bath or use as a soothing and relaxing body rub.

For a relaxing bath that is especially beneficial for swollen legs, add 1 drop each of chamomile and lavender oil to the bathwater after it has settled. Or ask your partner to gently massage your back with the following blend each evening before retiring.

### Evening Massage Oil Blend

*40 ml almond oil*
*5 ml avocado oil*
*5 ml wheat germ oil*
*8 drops geranium essential oil*
*8 drops lavender essential oil*
*4 drops chamomile essential oil*

Thoroughly blend all oils together and store in an airtight, amber-coloured glass bottle. Shake well before use.

## MORNING SICKNESS

To help overcome the problem of morning sickness and calm the stomach, place 1 drop of spearmint oil on your pillow each evening. On the floor beside your bed, place a bowl of boiling water to which has been added 6 drops of the same essential oil.

As you sleep, the calming fragrance of the spearmint oil will be inhaled, reducing the possibility of nausea and morning sickness.

## INSOMNIA

To relieve insomnia, try putting 1 drop of basil, chamomile, clary sage or lavender onto your pillow at night.

## STRETCH MARKS

A concern for all pregnant women is the legacy of stretch marks. To help prevent this problem it is essential to maintain the tone and elasticity of the skin by regularly massaging those areas where stretch marks are likely to occur: lower and upper abdomen, thighs and buttocks.

Massage these areas with the following oil blend.

### Anti-Stretch Mark Oil

*40 ml almond oil*
*5 ml avocado oil*
*5 ml wheat germ oil*
*5 drops carrot oil (available from health food stores)*
*8 drops tangerine essential oil*
*7 drops mandarin essential oil*

Thoroughly mix the oils together and store in an airtight, amber-coloured glass bottle. Shake well before use.

## CRACKED NIPPLES

This problem is more common than most people realise, and is even more likely to occur during breastfeeding. Apart from being extremely painful, there is also the possibility of infection. It is therefore important to take proper care of your nipples and to prevent this condition from occurring.

Apply the moisturising oil to your nipples after your bath or shower, massaging over the whole nipple and areola area. Start with the nipple, gently massaging each one by rolling it between a well-oiled thumb and forefinger for about 2 minutes. Then continue to gently massage the areola with well-oiled fingertips in small circular movements. The breasts can then be massaged as well (*see Breast Care*).

### Moisturising Oil for Cracked Nipples

*25 ml almond oil*
*20 ml apricot kernel oil*
*5 ml wheat germ oil*
*10 drops calendula essential oil*
*7 drops chamomile essential oil*
*8 drops rose essential oil*

Thoroughly blend all oils together and store in an airtight, amber-coloured glass bottle.

## VARICOSE VEINS

Varicose veins require professional treatment. However, in the early stages, gentle fingertip massage in the direction of the heart, and compresses, may help. When massaging the affected area of the legs, gentleness cannot be overemphasised: normal massage techniques can quite easily damage the fragile capillary walls.

Walking is also important, to prevent further congestion of the veins and to keep the blood circulating. Putting your feet up for an hour each evening after a footbath is also beneficial, as are a good diet and regular bowel movements.

### Finger Tip Massage Oil

27 ml hazelnut oil
3 ml wheat germ oil
20 drops geranium essential oil
10 drops cypress essential oil

Thoroughly blend all oils together and store in an airtight, amber-coloured glass bottle. Use within 2 months.

### Compress

4 drops geranium essential oil
2 drops cypress essential oil

Put the essential oils in a basin of hot water, sufficient to cover a compress. Soak the compress for 2 minutes, then squeeze it out until it stops dripping. Apply to the affected area and cover with plastic wrap and a pre-warmed towel. Leave on for at least 2 hours.

*See also Breast Care.*

# Prickly Heat

Prickly heat is a rash of tiny blisters that look like little red spots; it becomes extremely itchy. It can affect any part of the body and is caused by blocked sweat glands.

A warm bath, to which has been added 4 drops each of lavender and eucalyptus oil, is very soothing. Topical treatments include applications of aloe vera juice or gel, bicarbonate of soda and chickweed ointment *(see Chickweed Ointment)*.

*See also Aloe Vera, Itchiness, Skin Irritations.*

# Prostate Health

*See Zinc.*

# Protein

Protein is needed by our bodies for the building and replacement of cells and for the production of some enzymes and hormones. Proteins are comprised of amino acids, which are obtained from such sources as fish, meat, eggs, cheese, legumes, tofu and tempeh (fermented soya beans).

A well-balanced and carefully planned vegetarian diet that includes an adequate intake of vitamin B12 and iron is just as healthy as a meat-eater's diet. Protein in excess of our needs is not utilised by our bodies.

There are a number of factors which can greatly reduce the availability of dietary protein. If, for example, meat is the main source of protein, cooking it destroys at least one of the essential amino acids needed for building enzymes and healthy tissue. Additionally, liquids served with a meal delay protein digestion by reducing the concentration of gastric juices. Serving a concentrated protein food in the same meal with fats, sweets or starches can further inhibit digestion. Each of these foods requires different digestive juices, and when too large a quantity of concentrated food is eaten at a meal, much of it remains undigested.

Most people maintain health and adequate protein intake from a mixed, varied diet. A deficiency in one essential amino acid can be supplemented by adding another protein which contains the missing amino acid. However, there is no need to eat a complete protein mixture at any one meal. What is more important is your amino acid intake for the day, the week or the month.

For a vegetarian, tofu is an important source of protein. It contains 7.8 per cent protein, 65 per cent of which can be used by the body: 225 g of tofu can supply the same amount of useable protein (20 g) as 100 g of beef. Tofu also contains around one-quarter the calories/kilojoules of beef, and, more importantly, it does not contain any cholesterol.

It is very low in sodium, easily digested, and contains vitamin E and B group vitamins, phosphorus, chlorine, potassium, and more calcium than cow's milk.

When assessing your diet it is important to ensure that there is not an excessive intake of protein. Excessive protein can place stresses on your digestive system. This is particularly the case with red meat, which is difficult to digest. Excess protein can help form uric acid, which can contribute to gout, and since it is stored as fat, it can also contribute to obesity, heart diseases and other conditions.

You will find that the amount of protein you need will be directly related to your lifestyle — if you play a lot of strenuous sport, work in a hot environment where you perspire a lot, or are mentally or physically stressed, you will need more protein. Vegetarians also need to be mindful of their protein intake, as do children, adolescents, and pregnant and lactating women. Assess your dietary needs and protein intake with your health practitioner or dietitian.

# Psoriasis

Rub a few drops of jojoba oil into the affected area as needed.

*See also Eczema, Itchiness, Skin Irritations.*

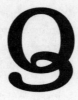

# Quassia

The quassias (*Quassia amara*) are native to South America and Jamaica. The chips, or wood shavings, have natural insecticide qualities which make them ideal for controlling many soft-bodied insects, such as head and pubic lice.

Some chemists may still stock quassia chips. If not, they can order them in for you; herbal suppliers, some health food or specialty shops may also be able to help.

To make a rinse for controlling head lice, boil 15 g of quassia chips in 2 litres of water in an enamel or stainless steel pan for 2 hours, topping up the liquid if necessary. Strain and add 1 tablespoon of cider vinegar to every 300 ml of liquid. Apply by combing through the hair with a very fine-toothed comb. Repeat at 2-week intervals, 4 times in total.

*See also Head Lice.*

# R

## Rashes

Itchiness from a nettle rash, a heat rash, an allergy rash or a rash that results from a viral infection may be relieved by a paste of bicarbonate of soda and water. Itchy heat rash can be relieved by soaking in a tepid bath in which ½ cup each of salt and vinegar has been dissolved.

Chickweed ointment will relieve most itchy rashes. To make your ointment, simmer 1 cup of fresh chickweed in ½ cup of olive oil for 30 minutes. Cool, strain and apply to the affected area as required.

Keep surplus lotion in an airtight, sterilised glass bottle for future use.

*See also Chamomile, Itchiness, Nettle Rash, Prickly Heat, Skin Irritations.*

## Raspberry Leaf

Raspberry leaf (*Rubus idaeus*) is accredited as a remedy for breaking up and aiding the expulsion of kidney and gall bladder stones, strengthening the uterus and entire reproductive system, coordinating uterine contractions and pangs in childbirth, and decreasing chances of miscarriage. Modern research has confirmed that one of its active constituents — fragrine — does actually improve the muscle tone of the uterus. Raspberry leaf is also an excellent remedy, when taken as a tea or enema, to treat flu and diarrhoea in children.

Raspberry leaf is available as a dried herb, as tablets, and as powdered herb capsules from health food stores.

# Relaxation

*See Stress and Tension.*

# Rejuvenation

We cannot recapture lost youth, but a proper diet, plenty of sleep, and regular intake of certain living foods will help our bodies generate young cells instead of old. Mung bean sprouts especially are excellent for the production of young cells; they should be eaten on a daily basis.

# Revitalisation

Revitalise yourself after a busy day, when you still have to go out at night, by adding 3 drops each of bergamot and ylang-ylang oil to a warmish bath and then soaking in it for 10 minutes. Unwind with a mixture of lavender and rosewood oil in your evening bath.

If your daily schedule doesn't always allow for a relaxing bath, you can still enjoy the benefits of fragrant oils in an aromatic shower. Mix 30 drops of your chosen oil with 40 ml of almond oil, dilute 50/50 with water, and rub this over your entire body. Plug the shower drain and sprinkle in some of the same aromatics as the water collects.

You can help revitalise your body and restore your health after illness by adding 6 drops of tangerine oil to your bath, or by adding the oil to a bowl of hot water and taking it as an inhalation. Tangerine oil is also good for a soothing back massage for anxiety or for expectant mothers — blend 3 drops of oil with 10 ml almond oil.

*See also Fatigue, Massage, Mental Fatigue, Thyme.*

# Rheumatism

Rub jojoba oil directly into sore joints whenever required. Because jojoba contains anti-inflammatory myristic acid, it has the potential to give relief.

There are also a number of fruits, vegetables and herbs which will prevent and relieve the discomfort of rheumatism. You must also abstain from foods which produce uric acid, such as eggs, legumes, nuts and seeds.

## DIET

▶ *Fruits:* Include all citrus fruits in your diet, as well as pineapple, figs, grapes, watermelon, nectarines, fresh cherries and strawberries. Drink citrus and pineapple juice daily.

▶ *Vegetables:* Eat artichokes, asparagus, celery, cucumbers, fresh young dandelion greens, garlic and lettuce. Celery is especially good for treating rheumatism, and can be eaten as often as you like.

▶ *Herbs:* Use licorice root, horseradish, dandelion root, yarrow, elder flowers, stinging nettle, feverfew, chickweed, meadowsweet, chamomile and parsley. Any of the herbs can be drunk as a tea 1 hour before meals. Meadowsweet is particularly soothing and anti-inflammatory, and may help with pain and inflamed joints.

## SWELLING AND PAIN

Chamomile, lavender and rosemary essential oils make excellent rubs for inflamed and painful joints. Dissolve 5 ml of any one of the 3 essential oils in 45 ml of olive oil, and store in an airtight, amber-coloured glass bottle. Use within 2 months.

Apply the lotion to inflamed joints whenever necessary.

## RHEUMATIC MUSCLES

Use the same essential oil lotion as recommended on previous page every 2 hours.

*See also Aching Joints and Muscles, Chamomile, Lemon Balm (Spirit of Balm), Sage.*

# Rhinitis

*See Hay Fever, Sinusitis.*

# Rosemary

Rosemary (*Rosmarinus officinalis*) is one of the famous herbs of folklore, and is known for making people more mentally alert. It is beneficial for the hair and scalp, as well as being a deodorant, a mouthwash and a bath herb. When included in bathwater it will stimulate the circulation, soften the skin, relieve stiff joints and relax aching muscles. The oil can be added to ointments for muscular aches and rheumatism, and can also be used as an antiseptic. Rosemary has a mildly anti-inflammatory effect on slow-healing wounds.

Dried rosemary and its essential oil are available from health food stores.

# S

## Sage

In the Middle Ages, when plants were considered much more remarkable than they are now, the common sage was believed to prolong life, heighten spirits, keep off toads, avert chills, and enable maidens to see their future husbands.
Today we know that this universal herb can be used as a hair rinse and tonic, a mouthwash to keep teeth white, and for rheumatism.

Rub a fresh sage leaf on your teeth and watch it take away the plaque! Taken as a tea it will help people who sweat too much, alleviate wind and cramps, strengthen the stomach, aid in the elimination of worms in children and dry up milk in nursing mothers. When used as a gargle it is a remedy for sore throat and laryngitis, and when blended with brandy or cider vinegar it makes an ideal mouthwash for sweetening the breath.

Cold sage tea can be used as an astringent tonic to help close large facial pores after cleansing; when used as a final hair rinse, it will stop your hair going grey.

### Oily Skin Tonic

Put 3 tablespoons of dried sage in a ceramic bowl. Mix 300 ml each of cider vinegar and distilled water in an enamel or stainless steel pan, then heat to just below boiling point. Pour the liquid over the herbs, cover tightly with plastic wrap and leave to steep for 12 hours. Strain and bottle for future use.
Gently dab on cleansed skin with a cotton ball, then leave to dry.
Finish off with a moisturiser.

# Salad

*See Energy Fruit Salad, High-Protein Mixed Salad.*

# Salt

Salt is one of the most commonly used food additives, but it can be dangerous to health if used excessively. It is an inorganic substance, and is not utilised by the body. It can cause stiffening of the joints, arthritis, hardening of the arteries and kidney disease. If it is taken in high enough concentrations, it will inhibit cell metabolism, and can eventually cause the death of cells.

The body only needs 0.5–1 g a day; this can be found naturally in fish, meat, vegetables and grains. Many people are consuming as much as 8–12 g of salt every day by eating fast or convenience foods, or adding salt to meals at the dining table. You should avoid salty foods such as crisps, pretzels and salted nuts, too much takeaway food, preserved meats, adding salt to your cooking, and putting the salt shaker on the table.

It is possible to buy many low-salt or salt-free foods, ranging from canned food, butter and margarine, bread, breakfast cereals and much more. Gradually using more of these types of food and adding herbs rather than salt to your cooking will help wean your tastebuds of salt. Many herbs will add flavours to your cooking that are very similar to salt.

## HERBAL SALT SUBSTITUTE

You can replace salt as a condiment with a mixture of herbs and other natural ingredients. This mixture will add flavour to your food as well as providing essential vitamins and minerals. But, like all condiments, the herbal substitute should be used with discrimination, so as to not overpower the natural flavour of the food.

All the ingredients needed to make your herbal substitute are readily available from health food stores.

Combine 1 tablespoon each of toasted sesame seeds and yeast flakes, 1 teaspoon each of dried and ground celery seed, oregano, thyme, garlic and coriander seed, and 3 strips of dried and ground lemon peel. For that salty taste, if you must have it, include a teaspoon of dried kelp. Mix these ingredients thoroughly, then reduce them to a powder in a blender or by rubbing them through a fine wire sieve. When mixed, store in an airtight jar. Label and date the jar and use the mixture within 12 months. It can be added to cooking and used at the table instead of salt.

# Salt Substitute

*See Salt (Herbal Salt Substitute).*

# Sandfly Bite

*See Insect Bite Itch, Stings and Bites.*

# Seasickness

Take about ½ teaspoon of powdered ginger about 30 minutes before sailing, or put a drop or two of ginger essential oil on a vitamin tablet and swallow.

# Sedative

Chamomile can be used as a mild sedative to help an active brain go to sleep, to ease menstrual cramps, or to help teething children.

Pour 100 ml of boiling water onto 10 g of dried chamomile flowers, infuse for 1 hour then strain. Reheat the tea and add honey to taste.

# Shingles

Apply apple cider vinegar to the affected area. Peppermint oil can also be used to soothe the discomfort. Dissolve 5 drops of peppermint oil in 15 ml of almond oil and apply liberally over the shingles.

A cup of nettle tea 3 times a day can also be helpful.

# Shower

*See Aromatic Shower.*

# Silicon

Silicon has been found to play an important role in preventive medicine, in particular controlling the diet. It is important for healthy fingernails and hair, and helps prevent calcium deposits around joints and further deterioration of arthritic conditions.

Natural food sources of silicon are apples (freshly picked only, not those kept in cold storage or the previous season's crop), apricots (fresh), asparagus, cabbage, carrots, celery, chives, cucumber, dandelion greens, lettuce (one of the best and most readily available sources), horseradish, lemon, oats, parsnips, potatoes, pumpkin seeds, rice (brown), spinach, strawberries, sunflower seeds, tomatoes and turnips.

# Sinusitis

With the arrival of spring, many people suffer sinusitis and hay fever. The traditional natural approach for relief is a combination of vitamins, minerals and herbs. In particular, vitamins C and A, zinc, and the herbs horseradish and fenugreek: vitamin C to reduce mucus, vitamin A and the mineral zinc to reduce susceptibility to infections and to increase the health of the epithelial tissue lining and sinuses, strengthening it against further attack from invading allergy proteins. Iron phosphate and potassium chloride also help reduce inflammation and mucus discharge.

The herbs horseradish and fenugreek are available as a supplement from health food stores. They will help remove mucus from your nasal and sinus passages, act a decongestant, soothe irritated nasal and sinus tissue and help dry up catarrh.

Include foods such as natural unprocessed bran, soya beans, oatmeal, raisins, sultanas, celery, cucumber, lettuce, cabbage, tomato, yellow vegetables, sprouted grains, green and red peppers, parsley and fresh fruit in your diet.

## INHALANT

Add 2 drops each of basil, eucalyptus, lavender and peppermint oil to a ceramic bowl containing 600 ml of boiling water. Sit with your face over the bowl and drape a towel over your head to form a tent — don't let the steam escape.

The inhalation procedure should not be used more than 3 times a day, and for no longer than 10 minutes each time. (People with heart and blood pressure problems, asthma or other breathing difficulties, broken skin or visible, dilated red veins should avoid using steam inhalations, unless otherwise directed by their health practitioner.)

## NASAL WASH

For those of you who don't mind minor momentary discomfort, a saltwater nasal wash gives quick relief to blocked sinus passages. Dissolve 1/4 teaspoon of salt in 1 cup of lukewarm water. Bend over a sink, hold the cup close to your nose with your left hand, close your right nostril with your right index finger and inhale the salty water into your left nostril. Spit the water out through your mouth. Swap hands and repeat the procedure with the other nostril.

## ALLERGY SUFFERERS

Cod liver oil is an old standby and natural food supplement. Taken as prescribed it will help allergy sufferers. However, always consult a health practitioner.

*See also Allergies, Hay Fever, Horseradish, Nasal Congestion.*

# Skin Care

Your skin is a living, breathing, eliminating and self-regenerating organ, and taking care of it correctly is very important. Before you start, however, you must learn to observe your skin's requirements, which will alter according to your state of health, your diet, and the climate in which you work and live.

The skin is made up of 3 distinct layers: the first, or lower level, is called the subcutaneous or basal layer. It is followed by the dermis, and then the epidermis. The subcutaneous layer contains muscles and fatty tissue; the sensory nerves, blood and lymph vessels, sebaceous glands and hair follicles are located in the epidermis. Skin cells are made in the dermis and travel up to the epidermis; in doing so, they constantly renew themselves.

Using essential oils and seed oils, such as almond oil, will help protect your skin against moisture loss and external damage, dirt and grime. Essential oils will penetrate to this bottom layer of skin, where they will exert their beneficial effects. Some oils will nourish the newly formed cells; others will help stimulate the cell-renewal process. It must be remembered, though, that these results will not be instantaneous; new skin cells can take 3–4 months to reach the epidermis.

Essential oils work to help slow the ageing process. Their nourishing and regenerative properties stimulate the rate at which new skin cells reproduce, reducing the time it takes for new skin growth and the removal of dead cells. At the same time, using essential oils will prevent congestion of the skin's eliminative process, speed up the removal of toxins, and improve circulation;

the oils also act as bactericides and anti-inflammatories and calm sensitive and damaged skin.

## MAINTAINING HEALTHY SKIN

Cleansing and moisturising will counteract the drying, chapping and roughening caused by the wind, sun and other environmental conditions, and help speed up the skin's renewal process. However, skin care products are not the only answer to skin problems, and they are by no means miracle products. A holistic approach, which includes regular exercise and a good diet, is also essential, to ensure that you have a well-balanced source of vitamins, minerals, herbs and amino acids. As well as being important to the functions of the body in general, vitamins B3, B5 and B6 are vital to the health of your skin. Zinc also plays an important role by assisting in the healing process and increasing your resistance to skin eruptions; vitamin A helps the skin retain moisture and keeps it in good condition; and vitamin C assists in the formation and elasticity of tissue, and in skin repair. They are available as supplements from health food stores but, where possible, it's better to get your daily intake of essential vitamins and minerals in a well-balanced diet.

Herbs and foods such as alfalfa, dandelion, burdock, parsley, sage, wheat germ, peanuts, brewer's yeast, unpolished rice and soya beans will help provide the essential B Group vitamins, and for vitamin C there is, of course, oranges. Green and red peppers are also a good source of vitamin C, as are Brussels sprouts, blackcurrant juice, watercress, dandelion greens and tropical fruits such as rockmelons, mangoes and pawpaws. Yellow and orange vegetables are a good source of vitamin A, as is sweet potato and herbs such as alfalfa, burdock, cayenne, dandelion greens, parsley and watercress. Dandelion has at least 4 times the vitamin A content of all other greens on the market. Zinc can be found in foods such as kelp, the herb marshmallow, oysters, lean beef, lean pork, brown rice, salmon, fish, crabs and lobsters.

# EXFOLIATING THE SKIN

Dust, dirt, pollution and inactivity will cause the pores of your skin to become clogged and congested. Daily body brushing (*see* **Dry Bathing**) is essential, to open your pores and to allow toxins to escape through increased lymph flow. In addition, exfoliation will remove dead, clogging cells, improve circulation, and leave your skin smooth, soft and glowing.

You can exfoliate while relaxing in an evening bath or in the shower. Add 2 tablespoons of medium ground oatmeal and 2 tablespoons of dried chamomile to a muslin bath bag. If you don't have a bath bag, place the ingredients in the centre of a square of muslin, draw up the sides and tie with a piece of ribbon. Oatmeal is a well-known skin softener, and as you rub your skin you will actually feel the impurities and rough skin float away.

Your elbows should be scrubbed daily with a soapy pumice stone (available from chemists), or a bath bag filled with the oatmeal mixture, until all ingrained dirt has disappeared. Next, bleach the reddened skin with lemon juice and then massage with a moisturising cream.

Friction massage your lower legs, thighs, upper torso and arms with a loofah during a warm bath or shower to accelerate cell metabolism and improve the circulation. Always massage upwards, in the direction of your heart.

Coarse sea salt on the loofah will help improve skin colour, and is excellent for clearing flaking skin and stubborn surface spots. Alternatively, friction massage with a bath bag filled with the oatmeal/chamomile mixture, then rinse off thoroughly and pat yourself dry with a towel.

Finish off the exfoliating process by massaging the following moisturising cream into your feet, legs, knees, arms and elbows. Smooth the cream firmly and upwards into your skin.

Melt together in a double stainless steel or enamel pan, over a low heat, 50 g of anhydrous lanolin (wool fat, available from chemists), 50 ml of olive oil and 25 ml of almond oil. Once completely liquid, pour the mixture into a sterilised airtight glass jar, and allow to cool.

# NOURISHING THE SKIN

To keep your skin looking healthy and supple, use a nourishing lotion regularly after your bath or shower.

A simple moisturising lotion can be made by blending together 50 ml of glycerine, 75 ml of rosewater, 45 ml of almond oil, 20 ml of wheat germ oil, 5 ml of jojoba oil, 12 drops of rose oil and 8 drops of oil of frankincense (optional). Place in an amber-coloured glass bottle, seal tightly, and shake well to thoroughly mix all ingredients.

Apply generously, massaging well into your skin.

# PROTECTION

Wind, cold weather, air conditioning and the sun can all dry and damage your skin. Protection is a must, and can be simply achieved with natural homemade preparations.

To stop your facial skin and hands becoming dry, scaly, chapped or split, apply the following moisturising lotion morning and night, or whenever required. It will keep your skin soft and supple.

Mix 20 g of ground almonds and 3 drops of pure rose oil with 500 ml of distilled water and allow to stand for 1 hour. Strain through fine muslin, add ½ teaspoon of sugar and 6 drops of friar's balsam (tincture of benzoin, available from chemists) and stir until the sugar has dissolved.

Bottle and seal.

# CHAPPED SKIN

For skin that is already chapped, make up the following oil and massage it over the affected area. Blend 10 drops of rose oil, 10 drops of chamomile oil, 5 drops of lemon oil and 5 drops of lavender oil with 30 ml of almond oil. Store in an amber-coloured glass bottle away from direct heat or sunlight, and use within 2 months.

Chapped and sore lips can be eased by applying a mixture of 2 drops of chamomile oil, 2 drops of geranium oil and 2 teaspoons of aloe vera juice (available from health food stores).

For cold sores, put 1 drop of either tea-tree or chamomile oil on a cotton bud and apply it directly to the sore as soon as it appears. Repeat every day.

## REJUVENATING LOTION

To make soothing and rejuvenating skin lotion, warm 1 cup of clear honey in a saucepan, then add ½ cup of milk and 2 teaspoons of rosewater, turning off the heat as you do. Stir the mixture thoroughly, allow to cool, then pour into a sterilised container and store in the refrigerator.

Before using, stir well, then pour a little of the lotion into a saucer. Soak cotton wool balls in the lotion and pat onto your face and neck every night. Do not rinse off until the following morning.

## SKIN CARE TIPS

▶ Be gentle when applying preparations; don't irritate or drag your skin.
▶ Smooth lotions and oils on, then blot off any excess after about 15 minutes.
▶ Avoid extreme heat or cold; both are bad for your skin.
▶ Clean your facial skin regularly.
▶ Don't overcleanse or clog your pores.
▶ Avoid harsh toning.

*See also Chamomile, Chapped Lips, Honey, Lavender, Sage.*

# Skin Irritations

In many cases skin irritations are caused by contact with a particular substance, such as strong or highly perfumed soap, washing powder and liquid, cheaper costume jewellery, cats, dogs, powder paints, cement, etc. Diet and stress can also aggravate skin complaints. Avoid cow's milk — goat's milk is an excellent substitute — and refined, processed foods. Eat plenty of wholemeal flour products, sprouts (especially mung beans and alfalfa), fresh fruit and vegetables, dried beans, lentils, soya beans, nuts, yeast, B vitamins, honey and sunflower and sesame seeds.

For general skin irritations apply aloe vera to the affected area, and drink aloe vera tea 3 times a day. Calendula lotion can be used as a soothing balm. To make your balm, put 2 tablespoons of dried calendula petals (available from most health food stores) and 5 tablespoons of glycerine in a small ceramic bowl. Place the bowl in a saucepan of boiling water and simmer over a low heat for 30 minutes. Remove from heat and strain. Discard the used petals and store the lotion in a sterilised, airtight glass bottle. Apply generously to the affected area as needed.

Tea-tree lotion (which is the most common way to purchase the oil) will give soothing relief to dry skin, cracked heels, sunburn and other skin irritations (including shaving rash, nappy rash and chafing). A few drops of jojoba oil applied directly to the affected area will also give relief and help moisturise your skin.

Cucumber is very soothing for inflamed and sore skin. Apply slices as needed directly on the affected area, or grate and massage the mixture well into the skin.

Psoriasis can be eased by rubbing a few drops of jojoba oil (pronounced ho ho ba, and available from health food stores and chemists) onto the affected area as needed.

Itchiness caused by a nettle rash, heat rash, allergy rash, or a rash that results from a viral infection may be relieved by a paste of bicarbonate of soda and water. Itchy rash can be relieved by soaking in a tepid bath in which ½ cup each of salt and vinegar has been dissolved.

---

*See also Aloe Vera, Chamomile, Eczema, Honey, Itchiness, Jojoba, Nettle Rash, Prickly Heat, Skin Care (Chapped Skin and Chapped Lips), Tea-Tree Oil.*

# Sleep

We all need regular, restful, natural sleep to keep healthy. Sleep allows the mind and body to unwind and restores lost energy. Yet all of us at some time have one of those nights where we just can't go to sleep. Fatigue, tension, anxiety, overexcitement or pain are some of the causes of an occasional sleepless night.

If you can't sleep, ask yourself why. Do you tend to overwork every day? Do you feel almost too exhausted to get ready for bed? If the answer is yes, you are creating a vicious circle of overtiredness: the inability to relax and regenerate at night causes you even more fatigue the next day, and so on. Re-examine your daytime activities and establish a natural rhythm that allows your body to relax.

Of course, overwork may not always be the problem. If you feel that your daily habits are not causing excessive fatigue but that you are still unable to have a restful night's sleep, look at your sleeping environment. Is your bed comfortable? Does your bed sag in the middle? Is your mattress rock hard? Are your bedclothes too heavy? All these factors can prevent you having a restful night's sleep.

Choose a bed that is comfortable, yet firm, and will provide adequate support for your spine.

Sufficient fresh air at night and an adequate diet are also important. Stuffy rooms will leave you feeling jaded in the morning; they will dehydrate your skin, and can cause an accumulation of fluid around your eyes, making them baggy when you awake. Also, check your diet. If you continually suffer from insomnia, you may not be getting sufficient vitamins and minerals. If your diet is not adequate, take a daily supplement to ensure a balanced calcium and magnesium intake. Include the following foods in your diet: apples, avocados, barley, almonds, cabbage, celery, sweet corn, lettuce, fresh mushrooms, onions, spring onions, green peas, baked potatoes, brown rice, soya beans and tomatoes.

Herbal teas which are soothing and strengthening to the nerves can be taken after dinner, instead of coffee, and $\frac{1}{2}$ hour before going to bed. Chamomile is an excellent choice; it will soothe your nerves and help promote sound, natural sleep.

When you finally retire, remove all external disturbances such as a ticking clock or a humming electrical machine. You could also try changing the light bulb in your bedside lamp to a low-voltage coloured one. Light shades of pink and certain tones of light green are excellent colours. Make sure you have good ventilation in your bedroom, because stuffiness is often the cause of waking in the night.

*See also Chamomile, Herbal Teas, Honey, Insomnia, Lavender.*

# Sleep Pillows

*See Insomnia.*

# Soap

*See Chamomile.*

# Sodium

Having sufficient free natural sodium in your diet can preserve suppleness and ease of movement and help keep the degenerative processes of old age at bay. However, it must be remembered that consumption of natural sodium does not mean the use of commercially available salt, or of the salt found in heavily processed foods — it means the intake of the mineral as it occurs naturally in food.

Just as phosphorous and calcium work hand in hand, so do sodium and potassium. If you haven't enough sodium in your diet you may suffer digestive problems, particularly those connected with incorrect functioning of the liver. Sodium also plays an important role in maintaining correct blood plasma levels, in the efficient removal of carbon dioxide, and in the absorption of calcium and magnesium salts.

Natural sources of sodium are brown rice, carrots, coconut meat and milk, celery, dandelion greens, dried fruits (apricots, figs, peaches, raisins), horseradish, kelp, olives, parsley, watercress, and most raw fruits and vegetables.

## Sore Throat

For a sore throat, add 4 drops of tea-tree oil to 25 ml of warm water and gargle 2 or 3 times a day.

Honey mixed with lemon juice will also soothe a sore throat. Take 1 teaspoon of the mixture every hour or so.

*See also Chilli, Sage.*

## Spasmed Muscles

*See Muscle Spasms.*

## Spearmint

Spearmint (*Mentha* x *spicata*) is one of the most commonly grown mints in the home garden, and until the seventeenth century was the most favoured of the mints for medicinal purposes. John Gerard, in his famous Herbal, says of its medicinal properties: *It is good against watering eies and all manner of breakings out on the head and sores. It is applied with salt to the bitings of mad dogs ... They lay it on the stinging of wasps and bees with good success.*

On hot, humid days spearmint makes a very refreshing drink. It has similar properties to peppermint; it will help dispel flatulence and prevent bad breath, is good for the gums, helps whiten teeth, and stimulates the digestive system. The calming fragrance of the pure essential oil will help reduce the possibility of nausea and morning sickness during pregnancy.

Both the essential oil and dried herb are available from health food stores.

# Spider Bite

*See Insect Bite Itch, Stings and Bites.*

# Splinters

Splinters can be extracted without pain by first applying olive oil to the affected area. Deep splinters can be removed by applying a castor oil poultice. It will draw out both the splinter and the infection.

# Sprains and Strains

For strained, sprained, stretched, twisted and torn ligaments (including wrenched ankles and twisted knees), massage the affected area with linseed oil every few hours when the pain is acute, then follow up with a daily massage of the area until it has completely recovered.

## SPRAINS, STRAINS AND SWELLINGS

Slices of onion warmed in hot water and applied as a poultice are effective as a first aid measure.

A compress of apple cider vinegar will reduce swellings. Dip a clean cloth into warmed vinegar, wring it out and apply it to the sprain as hot as can be tolerated. Change frequently. Once the swelling has gone down, massage the area well with a 50/50 mixture of rosemary essential oil and linseed oil.

## WRENCHED ANKLES

Massage with the rosemary/linseed oil mixture (*see above*).

## UNDERTONED MUSCLES

For undertoned muscles, weak and floppy muscles that suffer strains, massage with the rosemary/linseed oil mixture (*see above*). This mixture is also excellent for relieving tight muscles and muscles in spasm due to sporting activities (*see also **Muscular Aches and Pains***).

# MUSCULAR PAIN/SORE MUSCLES

*See Aching Joints and Muscles, Bathing, Chamomile, Lavender, Muscular Aches and Pains, Thyme, Witch Hazel Ointment.*

# Sprouts

*See Living Foods.*

# Stings and Bites

As a general first aid measure, apply the inside of a banana skin to the painful area, or split an aloe vera leaf (*Aloe barbadensis*) and rub the gel gently over the area.

Neat lavender oil applied to the site of a sting will also give relief. Apply 1 drop of oil, and then continue to apply 1 drop of oil every 5 minutes, or until it can be seen that the drop is being absorbed. Apply no more than 10 drops altogether.

You can also get quick relief from the pain of insect bites by applying eucalyptus oil to sore and swollen areas. Repeat if necessary.

## MOSQUITO AND ANT BITES

Mosquito and ant bites can be relieved by the application of bicarbonate of soda paste.

An application of neat lavender oil will also ease the itchiness of a mosquito bite. If you have been bitten over a large area, dilute 10 drops of lavender oil and 5 drops of thyme oil in 250 ml of cider vinegar and add this mixture to a warm bath. Afterwards, apply neat lavender oil to all the bites.

## BEE AND WASP STINGS

Bee and wasp stings can be relieved by applying a thick paste of bicarbonate of soda and then covering the affected area with a cold, wet cloth. (With a bee sting, you must first remove the actual stinger before treating with the soothing agent.) To remove the sting, apply a honey compress to the area. To make the compress, spread 1 teaspoon of honey on a piece of folded muslin or a handkerchief.

To draw the pain from a bee sting, immediately apply a slice of raw onion or a piece of ice to the affected area.

Wasp stings can be soothed by repeated applications of cider vinegar.

## BEDBUGS AND FLEAS

Bathe the bitten areas with an antiseptic wash made from a few drops of lavender or tea-tree oil in a cup of warm water, and then apply 1 drop of lavender oil.

## JELLYFISH

Wash the affected area as soon as practical with soap and water, and apply 1 drop of lavender oil, followed by an ice pack (or piece of ice).

## JIGGERS

Jiggers are minute insects which burrow under the skin (usually through your feet) to lay their eggs. This is usually followed by infection, with red lines appearing up the leg or swelling of the lymph glands. If there is swelling of the lymph glands, consult your health practitioner.

Dissolve 10 drops of essential oil of thyme in 1 teaspoon of vodka or brandy, or even methylated spirits, and apply it to the area every 3 hours for 1 day. Lavender oil can then be applied 3 times a day until the condition eases. Again, if the problem persists, see your health practitioner.

## MIDGE BITES

Dilute 3 drops of thyme oil in 5 ml of lemon juice and apply to the bites. This will stop the irritation.

## PLANT STINGS

Wash the affected area with soap and water as soon as possible, then apply a cold lavender compress. Add 10 drops of lavender oil to 100 ml of cold water, then soak a piece of cotton gauze or a clean handkerchief in the liquid. Remove the cloth and squeeze it gently until it stops dripping, and apply to the affected area. Renew as required.

If irritation doesn't cease within a few hours, or appears to be getting worse, contact your health practitioner.

## SANDFLY BITE

Apply lavender oil as soon as possible after the bite.

## SPIDER BITES (Non-venomous)

Dilute 3 drops of lavender oil and 2 drops of chamomile oil in 5 ml of vodka or methylated spirits, then apply to the bite 3 times over a day. If reddening persists, seek medical advice.

---

*See also Insect Bite Itch.*

# Stomach

When you're suffering from an upset stomach or feeling a little out of sorts, try a cup of ginger root tea; to settle an acid stomach, take 1 tablespoon of potato juice in a small glass of warm water. A grated raw apple will also ease general gastric disturbances.

To make hot ginger tea, use 1 tablespoon of fresh grated ginger root per cup of water and simmer in a covered enamel or stainless steel pan for 10 minutes. Strain, then sip slowly.

An upset stomach can also be calmed and indigestion eased by adding 1 drop of peppermint oil and a little honey to a glass of warm water and sipping slowly. It acts extremely quickly.

---

*See also Acidity, Herbal Teas, Indigestion, Jojoba, Medicinal Food, Overindulgence.*

# Stress and Tension

In today's hectic world, stress and tension can take a severe toll upon your health and wellbeing.

If you're working long hours, and are totally involved and absorbed with your job or career, it's more than likely that you'll feel tired and jaded, and have little enthusiasm for life. It's time to get out of the grind and routine and make some time for fun. Life should not be a merry-go-round of stress or a devastating experience; it should be a time of joy and fulfilment. But only you can make it like that.

 ▶ *Learn to like yourself.* To like yourself you must have a PMA — Positive Mental Attitude. It is important to make that conscious effort towards positivity and not get drawn into other people's misery. In other words, give bad news a wide berth. Avoid the company of complainers, and if you find yourself starting to whinge about something, just STOP and forget about it and your stress levels will drop straightaway.

 ▶ *Learn to defuse stressful situations.* Assertiveness courses are a great way to learn how to deal with people who are aggressive or too passive, and with difficult problems. Such a course will teach you how to have the courage to state what you want and still listen to the other person's point of view. You will find that you become more flexible in your attitude, and you won't be burdened with undue stress and worry.

 ▶ *Set aside a little time for yourself each day to do absolutely nothing, and learn to meditate (**see Meditation**).* Or why not join a meditation group? You will meet like-minded people and make new friendships, and learn how to how to use your spiritual strength to keep stress under control.

 ▶ *Don't keep your feelings bottled up inside you.* Share your feelings with a friend or partner.

 ▶ *And don't be afraid to cry* — it's a great tension reliever.

 ▶ *Make exercise a regular part of your daily regime.* Physical exercise is one of the best natural stress busters, and a great tension reliever. Whenever you feel tense, have a stiff neck or headache, or just feel completely tied up in knots after a day at work, go for a long brisk walk, play a game of squash, cycle, swim, or do something similarly active. Remember, any exercise will help you relax and release built-up tension. If you don't have the chance — for instance, if you're at the office — sit back and take a few deep breaths. Breathe in deeply through your nose and out again several times; this will help to calm you down. (Breathe in through your nose to the count of 4, hold for 4, breathe out for 4, hold for 4 and start again.)

▶ *Learn to relax your face.* Once it is relaxed, the rest of your body tends to follow. Do this by relaxing the lower jaw; every time you feel your teeth clenching just let go. Your forehead will then follow and you'll lose those wrinkles across your brow. Another way to ease those tense muscles is to gently rub a drop of eucalyptus oil into your forehead. Be careful not to go anywhere near your eyes.

▶ A few drops of lavender essential oil rubbed into your wrists or onto the nape of your neck also has a calming effect.

▶ Drink a relaxing cup of herbal tea, such as lemon balm, chamomile, peppermint or lemon verbena. Basil and borage tea is especially good for unwinding. Or make up the following rosemary tonic, and drink a wineglassful when needed. Bruise 4 sprigs of fresh rosemary and put them in a ceramic pot. Add 2 cups of white wine, cover, and leave to infuse for 2 days. Strain before drinking.

▶ Revitalise yourself after an extra-busy day by adding a few drops of ylang ylang and bergamot oil to a warmish bath and soaking in it for 10 minutes. Unwind with a mixture of lavender and rosewood oil in your evening bath.

▶ Don't forget about sleep. Our bodies need adequate uninterrupted natural sleep to function correctly and to renew cells and restore our nervous system. When we lack sufficient sleep, our skin becomes sallow and we develop dark circles under our eyes.

# DIET

Diet also plays an important role in treating this problem, and it should include bran, brewer's yeast, green vegetables (including dandelion greens), oats and oatmeal, passionfruit, peaches, sunflower seeds, tomatoes, vitamin B, wheat germ and yogurt.

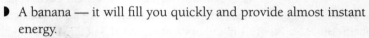

For an excellent source of vitamin B, and a great start to the day, nothing beats a good bowl of porridge with a few raisins and other dried fruit added. For a quick energy fix when you're feeling tired and slightly stressed out, try the following:

▶ A banana — it will fill you quickly and provide almost instant energy.
▶ A handful of sunflower seeds — high in B vitamins.
▶ Avocado and banana mashed up and mixed together with a little honey — serve this on oat biscuits for a powerful energy spread.

## STUDENTS

If you are a student feeling the stress of approaching exams, essential oils will help you cope and remain alert during long hours of study. Try any of the following. Simply add 1 drop of oil to one page in every book you are using.

▶ Basil — to clear the head.
▶ Bergamot — to bring freshness.
▶ Cardamom — to reduce mental fatigue.
▶ Lavender — ideal for physical and mental tension.
▶ Rose — to lift your spirits.
▶ Tangerine — energising.

*See also Chamomile, Fatigue, Floral Vinegar, Irritability, Massage, Mental Fatigue, Muscle Spasms, Nervous Tension, Revitalisation.*

# Stuffy Nose

*See Nasal Congestion, Vinaigrette.*

# Sulphur

Sulphur has a cleansing and antiseptic action on the whole of the digestive tract. It is needed for the formation of amino acids and the metabolism of proteins, and can be helpful with skin irritation conditions, especially those that do not respond to silicon.

Natural food sources are apples, asparagus, avocado, Brussels sprouts, cabbage, carrots, cauliflower, celery, cherries, cucumber, dandelion, eggplant, figs, grapefruit, horseradish, kelp, lettuce, mushrooms, onions (all members of this family, including brown and white onions, chives, garlic, leeks, shallots, and Welsh onions), oranges, pineapple, potatoes, pumpkin, radish, raisins, spinach, soya beans, strawberries, sweet corn, tomato, watercress and watermelons.

# Sunburn

If you suffer from sunburn it is important to drink plenty of fluids and herb teas, such as rosemary and lemon grass. To ease the stinging, soreness and pain, use any of the following first aid measures:

▶ Apply the juice straight from an aloe leaf to soothe and ease sunburn. Waterlily leaves and stems will also give relief.
▶ Dab milk onto affected area. Yogurt is also effective.
▶ Apply thin slices of cucumber to painful areas to ease stinging and give relief.
▶ Apply a paste of bicarbonate of soda to the affected area to give relief.

---

**Warning:** *Refer severe sunburn to your health practitioner.*

## SUNBURN LOTION

This lotion will ease mild sunburn and prevent further moisture loss from your skin.

*50 ml glycerine*
*40 ml aloe vera juice*
*10 ml wheat germ oil*
*10 ml jojoba oil*

Mix all the ingredients, then beat them vigorously until they are completely emulsified. Store the lotion in a bottle and seal tightly. Use generously on affected skin.

---

*See also Burns, Floral Vinegar (Sun Exposure), Honeysuckle (Honeysuckle Ointment), Jojoba, Sun Protection, Sunstroke, Witch Hazel Ointment.*

# Sunflower

Sunflower (*Helianthus annus*) oil is the richest and most beneficial of all the seed oils; it contains vitamins B, C, E and F, and is rich in protein. The extracted oil is both diuretic and expectorant, and will successfully treat coughs, colds and bronchial complaints. It acts as a digestive, aids the lungs, and is a blood purifier. Fresh flower petals blended with equal parts of fresh peppermint leaves makes an excellent tea.

Cold-pressed sunflower oil is available from health food stores.

# Sun Protection

Excessive, prolonged exposure to the sun is a major cause of skin cancer. Skin damage can occur after 12–20 minutes' exposure to sunlight. This 12–20 minutes can add up by just hanging out the washing or walking to the shops. So all-day outdoor gardening or leisure activities obviously means greater exposure to the sun's harmful rays.

It is essential to protect all exposed skin, especially your face, whenever you are in the sun by wearing appropriate clothing, a wide-brimmed hat and a suitable sunscreen. Reapply frequently if you are spending all day outside, and pay particular attention to your nose. A lip balm that will help block UV rays should also be applied frequently. (The nose, the lips and the delicate skin around the eyes are particularly vulnerable.)

Sunglasses are also a must when you are out in the sun. Without them you risk the possibility of eye strain in bright sunlight, and damage (and eventual wrinkles) to the delicate skin surrounding your eyes. Wear sunglasses that protect and fit over your eyes without leaving white areas. Remember, if you can see your eyes when you are looking in the mirror with your sunglasses on they do not give proper protection.

To prevent uncovered skin dehydrating and drying out, it is important to use a moisturiser before you apply your sunscreen. The following natural moisturiser is ideal for nourishing your skin and in helping prevent it drying out:

Melt 10 g of beeswax and 5 g of anhydrous lanolin (wool fat) — both available from chemists and health food stores — in a double enamel or stainless steel saucepan over a medium heat. When completely liquid, stir in 60 ml of almond oil, 5 ml of wheat germ oil, and 20 ml each of aloe vera juice and distilled water. Remove from heat, stir in 1 teaspoon of clear honey and pour into a ceramic bowl. Beat gently until the mixture is cool and has a creamy texture, adding 12 drops of lemon juice and 6 drops of tincture of benzoin (friar's balsam) once the mixture begins to cool. Store in a sterilised glass jar with a tight-fitting lid and use within 2 months.

Even when you are taking precautions, a day outdoors in summer can still leave your skin feeling hot and sticky. The following natural soothing lotion will cool and refresh your skin and help counteract the dehydrating effects of the sun.

Blend 50 ml each of rosewater and witch hazel (both are available from chemists) with 100 ml of distilled water. Store in a purse-size spray-mist bottle. Spray onto your skin as desired, avoiding contact with your eyes.

A fresh cucumber can also be used to cool hot and sticky skin. Cut a large cucumber into chunks, process in a food blender, wash affected body skin, then gently apply the cucumber lotion.

Cold chamomile tea or elder flower tea, used externally, is also an effective remedy for soothing and cooling the skin.

*See also Jojoba, Heat Exhaustion, Sunburn, Sunstroke.*

# Sunstroke

Symptoms of sunstroke are dizziness, headache, nausea and dryness and redness of the skin.

Apply cold water compresses, to which 2 drops of eucalyptus oil have been added, to the head, the nape of the neck, the chest and the back. Put the patient to bed and continue sponging with compresses for at least 24–48 hours.

No solid food should be taken during this time; the person should just drink plenty of water or unsweetened fruit juice. Have the patient drink 3 litres of water to which ½ teaspoon of salt per litre has been added.

*See also Floral Vinegar (Sun Exposure), Heat Exhaustion.*

# T

## Tea-Tree Oil

The antiseptic action of the oil of the tea-tree (*Melaleuca alternifolia*) is considered 10 times more powerful than carbolic acid — and yet in small doses it is non-poisonous to humans! Australian Aborigines have long made use of this native tree in their medications. Its anti-viral, anti-fungal and anti-bacterial properties make it useful in treating a whole range of first aid situations as well as other minor problems: infections, sunburn, acne, athlete's foot, toothache and pyorrhoea, to name but a few.

A bottle in the bathroom cabinet is a must for emergency first aid situations. Use it for the following:

▶ For abrasions, cuts and scratches, wash the wound thoroughly then apply 2–3 times a day with a clean cotton wool ball. Two or 3 drops in a bowl of warm water makes an excellent antiseptic wash.

▶ Dab a drop of oil on mosquito stings and other insect bites to relieve the itchiness and irritation.

▶ For temporary relief of muscular aches and pains. Blend 6 drops of oil with 10 ml of olive oil and apply before and after exercise. To make the oil extra penetrating, add 10 drops of avocado oil to the blend, mixing thoroughly. A teaspoon of oil added to a hot bath will also help relieve muscular aches and pains.

▶ To treat minor burns, first flush the affected area of skin with cold water, then apply the neat oil.

▶ Apply to cold sores as soon as they appear, and use 3–4 times a day for up to, but no more than, 5 days.

- Tea-tree lotion (which is the most common way to buy the oil) will give soothing relief to dry skin, cracked heels, sunburn and other skin irritations (including shaving rash, nappy rash and chafing). It also helps clear pimples and kills bacteria. Apply 3 times a day.
- If your sore throat persists, add 4 drops of oil to 25 ml warm water and gargle 2–3 times a day.

# Teeth

*See Mouth, Oral Hygiene, Sage.*

# Thirst

On hot summer days, instead of the traditional cuppa, add herbs to your favourite beverages for a refreshing, healthy change. Try tomato juice with oregano or basil, mineral water with rose geranium or lemon balm, or a refreshing iced herbal tea with tangy mint.

Herbal teas can be made from many different herbs and are readily available from both health food stores and supermarkets, sold singly and as blended teas. Use only a ceramic teapot for making your herbal teas, and sweeten them, if you like, with a little honey. Don't use aluminium or other metal teapots, as they can quite easily mar the brew.

Peppermint tea, which has a soothing, refreshing and delicately fruity taste, is served, very sweet, several times a day all over the Arab world. In our society it is recognised more for its medicinal qualities. However, on hot summer days it makes a very refreshing drink when served alone or blended with conventional tea. Another great summer refresher is a tea made with equal proportions of dried chamomile, linden leaves and passionflower.

My favourite thirst quencher is made from lemon balm or lemon grass leaves and served chilled. It's equally delicious when made from common garden spearmint. Add 1 teaspoon of dried herb, or 1 tablespoon of fresh herb, to every 300 ml of boiling water and allow to infuse for 5 minutes. Pour into a large jug and melt into it 2 tablespoonfuls of clear honey. Three-quarters fill the jug with ice cubes and place in the refrigerator until cold. Add 1 cup of freshly squeezed orange juice and ½ cup of fresh lemon juice, then garnish with a few fresh herb leaves.

Iced herbal teas can be drunk at any time during the day, and are particularly delicious when mixed with chilled mineral water or fresh fruit juice. Add a long, leafy stalk of the appropriate herb for added flavour. Prepare your tea as for the lemon balm thirst quencher. Try herbs such as chamomile, mint, marjoram, lemon verbena, or scented geraniums (*Pelargonium* spp.).

# Thyme

During the Middle Ages, thyme was given by a lady to her beloved knight as a farewell gift when he embarked on the Crusades. And those daring knights who ate thyme were thought to become more courageous.

Today we know that thyme is rich in thymol and has powerful antiseptic and cosmetic properties. It acts as an astringent, helping to clear spots and acne, and cleansing, soothing and refreshing the skin.

For a quick pick-me-up, try a cup of thyme tea, and hold a bunch of the fresh herb to your nostrils as well. Crush the herbs with your hand and breathe in their fragrance. Thyme tea also aids digestion and tones up the nervous system and respiratory organs; it is also reputed to alleviate the discomfort of a hangover. The cooled tea makes an excellent mouthwash for freshening the breath and is reputed to calm a cough and get rid of phlegm. You can make a tea by infusing a few sprigs of thyme in hot water, or use a herbal tea bag (available from health food stores and supermarkets).

The oil of this herb is one of the strongest antiseptics known, and is helpful in treating infected wounds and fungal problems such as athlete's foot.

To treat cuts, grazes, bites and scratches, wash the area carefully with a warm saline solution to which have been added 2 drops of thyme oil. For athlete's foot and nits make a tincture from the dried herb.

To make your tincture, cover 100 g of dried thyme with 2 cups of cider vinegar. Keep the mixture in a sealed jar and shake every day for 2 weeks. Strain and store the thyme vinegar in an airtight, sterilised bottle. Apply once a day for athlete's foot; for nits, comb through the hair and leave overnight, then reapply in 10 days.

At the end of a busy day, relax your feet by soaking them in a soothing thyme footbath. Add 5 drops of thyme oil and 1 cup of bicarbonate of soda to a large bowl of warm water. Mix well and soak your feet for 20 minutes.

If you have thyme growing in your garden, use it for your footbath. Add ½ cup of cider vinegar and 2 tablespoons of fresh thyme to 2 cups of water. Bring to the boil, then reduce heat and simmer for 5 minutes. Pour the liquid into a large bowl, cool until just bearable, then soak your feet until the water is cool.

Muscular aches and pains, including rheumatism, can be eased by relaxing in a thyme bath. Place a large handful of the dried herb in the centre of a square of muslin cloth, draw up the sides, tie with a ribbon and hang from the tap so that the hot water gushes through the bag as the bath fills.

*See also Antiseptic, Athlete's Foot, Cough, Cuts and Grazes, Feet, Hangover, Head Lice, Herbal Teas, Indigestion, Mouth, Muscular Aches and Pains, Oral Hygiene, Overindulgence, Revitalisation.*

# Tiredness

Lack of energy and continual tiredness are usually the result of a bad diet and a lack of correctly balanced vitamins and minerals, especially the mineral iron.

To ensure that you have that get-up-and-go, include the following in your diet: alfalfa and mung bean sprouts, apricots, dried beans, broccoli, freshly grated raw beetroot, capsicums, carrots, cauliflower, cabbage, honey, horseradish, lemons, lettuce, lentils, oranges, parsley, peaches, spinach, soya beans, sweet corn, sweet potatoes, sesame seeds, sunflower seeds and tomatoes.

Oatmeal is good iron food, and will give you a good start to the day. You can get your daily ration from your porridge, if that's what you prefer. Add fresh seasonal fruit and some wheat germ and you have a super get-up-and-go breakfast.

Energy-giving teas can be made from rosemary or alfalfa. Drink 1 cup 2–3 times a day.

# Tonics

Tonic herbs are essential for keeping your body in the peak of health, especially during times of illness, stress and anxiety, or after an overindulgence of any kind. These herbs are unique, because they tone the whole of your body, from the inner blood tissues to the muscles, from the organs to the outer skin.

Herbs that should be included in the diet are alfalfa sprouts, carrots, sunflower seeds, sesame seeds and fresh young dandelion greens. A number of herbal teas also act as tonics, exerting their beneficial effect on your body:

- Dandelion tea acts as a general tonic that fortifies the body systems and has a beneficial effect on the liver, kidneys and gall bladder. Drink 1 cup 3 times a day.
- Horehound tea helps with blood circulation. Take 1 cup 3 times a day.
- Rosemary tea is a general tonic that aids relaxation. Take a small glassful as needed.
- Carrot juice is an excellent all-round tonic; of all the juices it is the best balanced in vitamins and minerals. Take 1 small glassful daily on rising, but no more.

# Toothache

For temporary relief, apply 1 crushed clove or a little oil of cloves to the painful tooth, or plug the cavity with cotton wool soaked in the oil.

Persistent toothache needs the prompt attention of a dentist.

# Trace Minerals

Most of the trace minerals seem to appear in the glandular system, and the part they play in good health is not yet fully understood.

# Travel Sickness

To help ease travel or motion sickness, chop up ½ teaspoon of fresh ginger, dust with powdered cinnamon and bind with honey. Take before a journey, and when symptoms occur. A few drops of peppermint or lavender oil added to a handkerchief or tissue and inhaled will also ease the nausea associated with travel sickness.

If you suffer from sea, car and air sickness, avoid sweet and starchy foods on the day of travel. Eat fruit or drink pure, unsweetened fruit juice only.

# U

## Ulcers

### MOUTH ULCERS

*See Mouth.*

### PEPTIC ULCERS

Drink 1 cup of alfalfa tea 3 times a day, or 1 cup of ginger root tea before meals, or as needed.

Eating a small piece of raw potato, about the size of a marble, before each meal will eliminate pain and help heal an ulcer.

*See also Acidity.*

## Underarm Deodorant

*See Hygiene.*

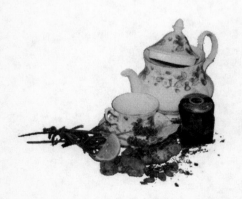

# Urinary Disorders

Your diet should include cabbage, mustard greens (very quick and easy to grow at home in pots), zucchini, squash, watermelon, spinach, raw beetroot (1 glass of juice morning and night), asparagus, green peppers, orange juice (freshly squeezed), watercress and fresh tomatoes (home-grown are best).

The following herbal teas will also help bladder problems:

▶ Bladder infection — drink 1 cup of parsley tea 3–6 times a day.
▶ Bladder weakness — drink 1 cup of yarrow tea 2–3 times a day, or as needed.

*See Cystitis, Kidneys, Medicinal Food (Barley).*

# V

## Vaginitis

*See Bathing, Soda Baths, Yeast Infection.*

## Valerian

Taken as a tea Valerian (*Valeriana officinalis*) is a remedy for insomnia, nervous disorders and pain, without being habit forming. It has a remarkable tranquillising effect, similar to Valium, and should be taken just before going to bed. Valerian tea will stop menopausal headaches. It is available as a dried herb from health food stores.

*Note: Valerian can act as stimulant rather than a sedative with some people. Although this is rare, if you have not previously tried this herb, start with a low dose to ascertain how it may affect you. It must not be used during pregnancy.*

## Varicose Veins

*See Pregnancy (Varicose Veins).*
*See also Feet.*

## Vinaigrette

A vinaigrette is no more than a strong-scented herbal vinegar, usually kept in a special 'smelling bottle'. They were extremely popular in Regency England, being considered an essential accessory for fashionable young men and women meeting in crowded ballrooms and stuffy taverns.

Today a vinaigrette makes an ideal natural addition to the bathroom cabinet to relieve a stuffy nose or headache. A vinaigrette can be made as follows:

*2 tablespoons dried lavender*
*2 tablespoons dried rosemary*
*1 tablespoon dried mint*
*1 tablespoon dried marjoram*
*150 ml cider vinegar*
*150 ml distilled water*
*1 teaspoon camphorated oil (available from chemists)*

Put all the herbs in a ceramic bowl. Combine the cider vinegar and distilled water, and heat in an enamel pan to just below boiling point. Pour the liquid over the herbs, cover tightly with plastic wrap and leave to steep for 24 hours. Strain, add the camphorated oil and mix well.

Push a small piece of natural sponge into a bottle. Pour in the vinegar liquid and seal tightly. Any leftover vinaigrette can be bottled and used in the bath or given to friends as a gift.

To use, remove the lid and hold the bottle under your nose. Breathe deeply to revive yourself if you are feeling faint, or to clear a stuffed-up nose.

---

*See also Nasal Congestion.*

# Vitality

We are always seeking ways to improve our health. The first step is a resolve to bring balance into your life — in other words, be good to yourself to maintain a healthy lifestyle.

▶ *Get Enough Sleep* — late nights and excessive lifestyles play havoc on the internal body systems, and eventually affect the way we look and feel. The body needs sufficient sleep to allow itself to regenerate. An inadequate diet will also affect our sleep patterns, especially if there is an insufficient vitamin and mineral intake.

Check your calcium and magnesium intake, make sure you get enough fresh air at night, and choose a bed that is comfortable, yet firm, and that will provide adequate support for your spine.

▶ *Exercise Regularly* — this is a must, as it promotes better circulation, deep breathing, and a healthier, more vibrant you. The correct use of muscles can reshape the body; it can lift sagging cheeks, melt away double chins, middle-age spread and abdominal bulges, restore elasticity to the skin, making it smooth and healthy, and iron out wrinkly necks and eliminate flabbiness.

▶ *Eat Plenty of Fresh Fruit and Vegetables Daily and Eat Less Fat* — good food is vital for good health. A properly nourished body should glow with the bloom of health. Deprive your body of essential nutrients over a long enough period and something, somewhere, will go wrong.

Eat vegetables every day, raw when possible. If they have to be cooked, use the microwave, or just steam or bake them until tender. Potatoes, and other roots, can be cooked in about 6 mm of water in the bottom of a glass baking disk at 180°C for 1½ hours.

▶ *Drink Plenty of Water* — water is essential to good health, to flush toxins from the body. Drink at least 8 glasses each day, preferably water that is free of chemical treatment (such as chlorine and fluoride). Natural mineral water closely resembles the water in your body and should be drunk in preference to town tap water.

▶ *Take Time to Relax* — learn to cope with stress and take time to relax. Exercise is one of the best natural stress busters. Go for a long walk, cycle or swim — any exercise will help you relax and release built-up tension. If you're unable to exercise take deep breaths to calm down — breathe in through your nose to the count of 4, hold for 4, breathe out for 4, hold for 4 and start again.

▶ *Learn to Meditate* — join a meditation group. You will meet like-minded people and make new friends, and you'll learn how to use your spiritual strength to keep stress under control.

Remember, though, too much of something can be just as unhealthy as too little of anything — concentrate on the overall picture for a healthier, vibrant you.

*See also Eating for Health and Energy, Exercise, Sleep, Stress and Tension, Water.*

# Vitamins

Confusion about the variety and multiplicity of vitamins available from chemists and health food stores may lead you to buy too many, too few, or products that are totally unsuitable for your needs.

Multivitamin capsules are rarely the answer: each individual's needs are so different that you still could find yourself lacking in some essential vitamins.

Vitamins are the building blocks that make us healthy, bounding-with-energy human beings. Select foods and herbs that contain the vitamins you need, and include them in your diet each day. Remember, natural sources are always better than pills.

Vitamin D is the only vitamin which is manufactured by your body; the rest must be absorbed from the food and drink you consume. Nearly all vitamins are manufactured by plants — a very good reason why you should eat plenty of fresh and chemical-free vegetables and herbs. A correct vitamin balance means good health both internally and externally: when you feel good, you look good.

## VITAMIN A

This vitamin cures skin diseases. Sources of vitamin A include yellow and orange vegetables, sweet potato, alfalfa, cayenne, dandelion greens, parsley and watercress.

## B GROUP VITAMINS

These vitamins calm the nerves and ensure good health of the nervous and digestive systems, regulate and stabilise liver function, convert unsaturated fats into body fuel, protect natural hair colour, prevent premature greying, are useful in skin disorders and help soften wiry or tightly curled hair, making it more manageable. Sources of B group vitamins include brewer's yeast, cheese, dandelion, eggs, legumes, milk, nuts, peanuts, potatoes, rice bran, soya beans, strawberries, unpolished rice, wheat germ and whey.

## VITAMIN C

This vitamin controls the tone and resilience of your body's cells, assists in repairing and renewing cells, and hardens the dentine of your teeth. It also carries hydrogen around the body, assisting with proper absorption of iron. Sources of vitamin C include Brussels sprouts, citrus fruits, fresh red cabbage, green and red peppers, guava, kale, mangoes, mustard greens, parsley, rockmelon, rosehips and sweet potato.

## VITAMIN D

This vitamin enables calcium and phosphorus to be used by your body, regulates your metabolism, and is necessary for the health of your eyes. We rely upon the sun for our intake of vitamin D.

## VITAMIN E

Vitamin E improves overall health and protects other vitamins from being oxidised, so that they are completely assimilated by the body in their pure state. Sources of vitamin E include wheat germ (the best and most available source), beans, peas, pumpkin seeds, oatmeal, safflower oil, soya oil and sunflower seeds.

## VITAMIN F

This vitamin controls your metabolic rate, takes care of your cholesterol balance, and prevents eczema and dull, dry hair. It also plays a role in the correction of dandruff and acne, and regulates overactivity of the sebaceous glands. Sources of vitamin F include seafood (tuna, salmon, eel), most nuts (except cashews), rice, vegetable oils and wheat germ.

## VITAMIN K

Essential for the blood's clotting action. Sources of vitamin K include: green leafy vegetables such as spinach, cabbage, carrot tops and alfalfa, and soya bean and cod liver oil.

## VITAMIN P

Rutin, the major part of this vitamin, keeps blood vessels pumping efficiently, and has great therapeutic value for infections and diseases of the eye. Sources of vitamin P include buckwheat and the pulp (not just the juice) of lemons and oranges.

## VITAMIN U

Occurs naturally in cabbage. Used to sooth irritation from peptic ulcers.

# Vomiting

To ease vomiting, take frequent sips of strong, hot peppermint tea. Prepare the tea using 3 or 4 peppermint tea bags (available from health food shops and supermarkets) to 1 cup of hot water. Infuse for 5 minutes and reheat if necessary.

---

*See also Nausea.*

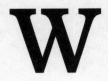

# W

## Warts

Never attempt to cut warts or dig at them and pull them off — it will just make matters worse.

There are a number of natural remedies which may prove successful, but they must be used continually if they are to work.

▶ Rub freshly crushed marigold leaves onto warts morning and night until they disappear, or squeeze a few drops from the hollow stem of a dandelion straight onto them. Repeat either procedure until they disappear.

▶ Apply the juice from the stem of the herb greater celandine. Take care to apply it only to the wart. If it touches healthy skin, immediately wash it off — if it is allowed to remain it will peel the skin off. Leave the wart uncovered and apply the juice morning and night. Within a fortnight the wart should have flaked away, leaving only healthy skin behind.

▶ In spring, drip the white sap from a dandelion stem onto the wart. On the two occasions that my son had warts on his fingers, this treatment was undeniably successful, with the warts disappearing after about 6 days.

▶ Other natural remedies are to apply the following directly onto the wart, at regular intervals: cabbage leaf juice, fresh pineapple juice or wheat germ oil.

## PERSISTENT WARTS

Put a drop of jojoba oil on the wart morning and night.

*See also Dandelion, Jojoba.*

# Wasp Sting

*See Insect Bite Itch, Stings and Bites.*

# Water

Every living organism on this planet must have water to live, or the moisture in the air from water vapour. Without water we will dehydrate and die! However, pure, unadulterated water is a very rare commodity in today's world. Yet it is one of the vital ingredients in maintaining our health.

So what do we do to overcome this problem? Water does not necessarily need to be drunk from a glass; there is enough to sustain us in the skins of fresh fruit and vegetables, if we eat enough.

If human beings were able to maintain an ideal diet it would be 80 per cent fresh fruit and vegetables, and we would rarely require supplementary liquids. However, an ideal diet, like pure water, is very rare in our modern society.

For a small investment you can purchase a water filter. Most of them, however, are incapable of making our supplied water safe for drinking. Cheap filters usually only remove dirt particles. The expensive counterparts can do a great deal more, including sterilising the water with an ultraviolet light beam. However, the better the filter the more it will cost you.

Boiling drinking water only kills fungus or bacteria which have succeeded in beating the chemicals used at the water treatment works. In fact, boiling water that has been treated with fluoride only tends to increase the concentration of fluoride in the water. And collecting rainwater, especially in city areas, is little better. With so much pollution from industry, motor vehicles, power generation, etc., it would need to rain steadily for a number of days before the water could be considered safe to collect. Even then, this would only be in outer-city and rural areas.

We can obtain the pure water we need by eating more fresh fruit and vegetables, or by drinking their extracted juices. In addition to fruit and vegetable juices, we can make our own biochemical-free water easily and quickly. The first step is to sprout some wheat seeds.

Soak 1 or 2 tablespoons of seed in a large jar of water overnight. Drain and rinse 3 or 4 times. Place the jar in a dark cupboard, rinsing 4 or 5 more times a day, until the grass shoots begin to develop. Move the jar to a sunny spot, continue to rinse, and wait until the grass turns green. Cut off the growing tips of the shoots and add to a container of water. After about 20 hours, remove the shoots and you will have pure water, tasting unlike water you have ever tasted before. It is free of any polluting substances.

## ESSENTIAL WATER FACTS

▶ Water is the second most important element required for living. The most important is air.

▶ The adult body is 60–70 per cent water. Water is vital for the chemical reactions that occur in the body. It carries nutrients and oxygen to the cells, lubricates the joints and helps keep the body cool through perspiration.

▶ You should drink 8–10 glasses of water a day. This may seem a lot, but you should remember that you lose at least 2–3 litres of water from your body a day, and this must be replaced. Of course the more active you are the more water you lose, and therefore the more you need to replace.

▶ Water can be replaced by eating fresh raw fruit and vegetables, especially those with a high water content, and by drinking fruit juices, soup and soft drinks. Or, best of all, drink plenty of your own biochemical-free water. Plain water is the liquid that is most efficiently absorbed by the body.

▶ Caffeinated drinks, such as coffee, are not good replacement fluids, as caffeine causes you to lose even more fluid. Alcohol has the same effect.

▶ Feeling thirsty is your body's way of telling you that you are running low on fluids.

# Water Retention

Include plenty of apples, asparagus, celery, parsley and raw onion in your diet, plus grapes, pawpaw, strawberries and watermelon, when in season.

A cup of parsley, celery or fennel tea 1 or 2 times a day is also helpful.

## Wild Herb Garnish

*See Cooking with Herbs (Wild Herbs, Wild Herb Garnish).*

## Wild Herbs

*See Cooking with Herbs (Wild Herbs).*

## Wild Herb Salad

*See Cooking with Herbs (Wild Herbs, Wild Herb Salad).*

## Witch Hazel Ointment

Use this soothing cream to ease aches, sprains and sunburn.

*10 g beeswax*
*20 ml witch hazel solution (available from chemists)*
*20 ml rosewater*
*5 ml almond oil*
*60 ml hazel nut oil*
*6 drops tincture of benzoin (friar's balsam, available from chemists)*

Melt the beeswax in a double boiler (enamel or stainless steel) over a medium heat. When completely liquid, add the witch hazel, rosewater and oils, stirring until completely blended and liquid. Remove from heat, allow to cool slightly, add the tincture of benzoin, and beat with a wooden or electric mixer until cool and of a creamy texture. Store in an airtight, sterilised glass jar.

*See also Aches and Pains, Strains and Sprains, Sunburn.*

# Worms

The threadworm, which looks like tiny threads of dirty white cotton, is the one most commonly found in humans. It lives in the intestines and multiplies by crawling out, usually at night, and laying its eggs around the anus, hence the itching.

To avoid threadworms, your diet should include apples, cabbage, capsicums, figs, garlic, horseradish, onions, peaches, pineapple, pomegranate, pumpkin seeds, rhubarb, sesame seeds and sweet basil.

Anyone with worms should eat 6 pumpkin seeds as soon as they get up in the morning every day for 10 days and drink 1 cup of chamomile tea 3 times a day.

A grated raw carrot and 3 garlic cloves, eaten first thing in the morning on an empty stomach, will also help expel worms.

# Wrenched Ankles

*See Sprains and Strains.*

# Writer's Cramp

Anyone who has to hold their hand and forearm in one position for a long time can suffer writer's cramp.

Massage is the best immediate solution, but increasing your vitamin D and calcium intake also helps.

Make your own massage oil by dissolving 30 drops of either rosemary or geranium essential oils and 5 ml of wheat germ oil in 25 ml of almond oil. Store in an airtight, amber-coloured glass bottle, and use as required.

# Y

## Yarrow

Yarrow (*Achillea millefolium*) is an astringent and cleansing herb as well as being a styptic (a substance that will stop bleeding). It can be used in face masks, face scrubs, toners for large pores and overactive sebaceous glands, shampoos and mouthwashes. However, don't use it on the face by itself — a general wash or lotion made with yarrow may cause sensitivity to sunlight. When taken as a tea it is a good remedy for severe colds, especially when blended with equal quantities of peppermint and elder flower. Yarrow tea is a traditional remedy for kidney and liver diseases, bladder weakness, and catarrh of the air passages. It is also a remedy for teething, cramps and bed-wetting in children.

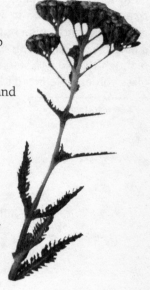

An ointment made from fresh yarrow leaves and olive oil is a traditional Scottish highlanders' remedy for bleeding and itchy piles, and it is also useful for healing cuts and wounds. The Norwegians use a tincture, made from the flowers, to relieve the pains of rheumatism. Because yarrow is rich in chlorophyll, it exerts a cleansing action on all the blood vessels, and is reputed to rectify high blood pressure.

Dried yarrow leaves are available from health food stores.

# Yeast Infection

An effective natural remedy for yeast infection in women is to apply fresh, natural yogurt inside the vagina 1 or 2 times a day. If symptoms persist, consult your health practitioner.

To treat yeast infections in babies and children, wash the affected area with garlic water, then gently apply garlic oil. Again, a health practitioner should be consulted if symptoms persist.

To make garlic water, chop up 2 cloves of garlic and steep in a covered ceramic bowl in 300 ml of hot water. Cool and strain.

To make garlic oil, chop up 6–12 gloves (depending on desired strength), combine with 500 ml of sunflower oil in a glass jar and seal tightly. Allow to stand for 14 days, then strain into an airtight glass bottle. Store in a dark, cool place.

*See also Garlic.*

# Z

## Zinc

Zinc deficiencies have been linked to male and female infertility, susceptibility to infection, behavioural and sleep disturbances, white spots on nails and slow wound healing. Good natural sources of this mineral are fish, lean meat, green leafy vegetables, pulses, nuts and wheat germ. Zinc citrate in tablet form is also available.

Growing your own organic vegetables is a big plus, as they contain more zinc than those grown with the help of chemical fertilisers. If it is not possible to grow your own, seek out a reliable retail supplier of organic produce.

Maintaining correct zinc levels in the body helps decrease cholesterol deposits, preserves the sense of taste, helps ensure fertility, and, in men, keeps the prostate gland healthy.